OPPOSING VIEWPOINTS® SERIES

Vaccines

I0811246

Other Books of Related Interest

Opposing Viewpoints Series

Big Pharma and Drug Pricing
COVID-19 and the Changing Way We Live and Work
QAnon and Other Conspiracy Theories
Trumpism and the Future of the Republican Party

At Issue Series

COVID-19 and Other Pandemics
The Role of Religion in Public Policy
The Role of Science in Public Policy
Vaccination

Current Controversies Series

Attacks on Science
Climate Change and Biodiversity
The Politics and Science of COVID-19
Universal Health Care

> "Congress shall make no law … abridging the freedom of speech, or of the press."
>
> *First Amendment to the U.S. Constitution*

The basic foundation of our democracy is the First Amendment guarantee of freedom of expression. The Opposing Viewpoints series is dedicated to the concept of this basic freedom and the idea that it is more important to practice it than to enshrine it.

OPPOSING VIEWPOINTS® SERIES

Vaccines

Lisa Idzikowski, Book Editor

GREENHAVEN PUBLISHING

Published in 2023 by Greenhaven Publishing, LLC
2544 Clinton Street,
Buffalo NY 14224

Copyright © 2023 by Greenhaven Publishing, LLC

First Edition

All rights reserved. No part of this book may be reproduced in any form without permission in writing from the publisher, except by a reviewer.

Articles in Greenhaven Publishing anthologies are often edited for length to meet page requirements. In addition, original titles of these works are changed to clearly present the main thesis and to explicitly indicate the author's opinion. Every effort is made to ensure that Greenhaven Publishing accurately reflects the original intent of the authors. Every effort has been made to trace the owners of the copyrighted material.

Cover image: Bangkok Click Studio/Shutterstock.com

Library of Congress CataloginginPublication Data

Names: Idzikowski, Lisa, editor.
Title: Vaccines / Lisa Idzikowski, book editor.
Description: First edition. | New York : Greenhaven Publishing, 2023. | Series: Opposing viewpoints | Includes bibliographical references and index. | Contents: Vaccines | Audience: Ages 15+ | Audience: Grades 10-12 | Summary: "Anthology of essays accompanied by original introductory material that explores the controversies surrounding the issue of vaccines in American society"-- Provided by publisher.
Identifiers: LCCN 2022021874 | ISBN 9781534509085 (library binding) | ISBN 9781534509078 (paperback)
Subjects: LCSH: Vaccines--Juvenile literature. | Vaccines--Social aspects--Juvenile literature. | Vaccination--Social aspects--Juvenile literature.
Classification: LCC RA638 .V3334 2023 | DDC 615.3/72--dc23/eng/20211220
LC record available at https://lccn.loc.gov/2022021874

Manufactured in the United States of America

Website: http://greenhavenpublishing.com

Contents

Chapter 3: Does Politics Alter the Perception of Vaccines in Society?

Chapter 4: What Is the Future for Vaccines?

The Importance of Opposing Viewpoints

Perhaps every generation experiences a period in time in which the populace seems especially polarized, starkly divided on the important issues of the day and gravitating toward the far ends of the political spectrum and away from a consensus-facilitating middle ground. The world that today's students are growing up in and that they will soon enter into as active and engaged citizens is deeply fragmented in just this way. Issues relating to terrorism, immigration, women's rights, minority rights, race relations, health care, taxation, wealth and poverty, the environment, policing, military intervention, the proper role of government—in some ways, perennial issues that are freshly and uniquely urgent and vital with each new generation—are currently roiling the world.

If we are to foster a knowledgeable, responsible, active, and engaged citizenry among today's youth, we must provide them with the intellectual, interpretive, and critical-thinking tools and experience necessary to make sense of the world around them and of the all-important debates and arguments that inform it. After all, the outcome of these debates will in large measure determine the future course, prospects, and outcomes of the world and its peoples, particularly its youth. If they are to become successful members of society and productive and informed citizens, students need to learn how to evaluate the strengths and weaknesses of someone else's arguments, how to sift fact from opinion and fallacy, and how to test the relative merits and validity of their own opinions against the known facts and the best possible available information. The landmark series Opposing Viewpoints has been providing students with just such critical-thinking skills and exposure to the debates surrounding society's most urgent contemporary issues for many years, and it continues to serve this essential role with undiminished commitment, care, and rigor.

The key to the series's success in achieving its goal of sharpening students' critical-thinking and analytic skills resides in its title—

Opposing Viewpoints. In every intriguing, compelling, and engaging volume of this series, readers are presented with the widest possible spectrum of distinct viewpoints, expert opinions, and informed argumentation and commentary, supplied by some of today's leading academics, thinkers, analysts, politicians, policy makers, economists, activists, change agents, and advocates. Every opinion and argument anthologized here is presented objectively and accorded respect. There is no editorializing in any introductory text or in the arrangement and order of the pieces. No piece is included as a "straw man," an easy ideological target for cheap point-scoring. As wide and inclusive a range of viewpoints as possible is offered, with no privileging of one particular political ideology or cultural perspective over another. It is left to each individual reader to evaluate the relative merits of each argument—as he or she sees it, and with the use of ever-growing critical-thinking skills—and grapple with his or her own assumptions, beliefs, and perspectives to determine how convincing or successful any given argument is and how the reader's own stance on the issue may be modified or altered in response to it.

This process is facilitated and supported by volume, chapter, and selection introductions that provide readers with the essential context they need to begin engaging with the spotlighted issues, with the debates surrounding them, and with their own perhaps shifting or nascent opinions on them. In addition, guided reading and discussion questions encourage readers to determine the authors' point of view and purpose, interrogate and analyze the various arguments and their rhetoric and structure, evaluate the arguments' strengths and weaknesses, test their claims against available facts and evidence, judge the validity of the reasoning, and bring into clearer, sharper focus the reader's own beliefs and conclusions and how they may differ from or align with those in the collection or those of their classmates.

Research has shown that reading comprehension skills improve dramatically when students are provided with compelling, intriguing, and relevant "discussable" texts. The subject matter of these collections could not be more compelling, intriguing, or urgently relevant to today's students and the world they are poised to inherit. The anthologized articles and the reading and discussion questions that are included with them also provide the basis for stimulating, lively, and passionate classroom debates. Students who are compelled to anticipate objections to their own argument and identify the flaws in those of an opponent read more carefully, think more critically, and steep themselves in relevant context, facts, and information more thoroughly. In short, using discussable text of the kind provided by every single volume in the Opposing Viewpoints series encourages close reading, facilitates reading comprehension, fosters research, strengthens critical thinking, and greatly enlivens and energizes classroom discussion and participation. The entire learning process is deepened, extended, and strengthened.

For all of these reasons, Opposing Viewpoints continues to be exactly the right resource at exactly the right time—when we most need to provide readers with the critical-thinking tools and skills that will not only serve them well in school but also in their careers and their daily lives as decision-making family members, community members, and citizens. This series encourages respectful engagement with and analysis of opposing viewpoints and fosters a resulting increase in the strength and rigor of one's own opinions and stances. As such, it helps make readers "future ready," and that readiness will pay rich dividends for the readers themselves, for the citizenry, for our society, and for the world at large.

Introduction

> *"Immunization prevents deaths every year in all age groups from diseases like diphtheria, tetanus, pertussis (whooping cough), influenza and measles. It is one of the most successful and cost-effective public health interventions. An additional 1.5 million deaths could be avoided, however, if global vaccination coverage improves."*
>
> *—World Health Organization, 2022*

Illness, disease, vaccines, and the controversy surrounding them, are nothing new. Over two thousand years ago, a deadly infectious disease, smallpox, caused untold numbers of people to suffer and die around the world. Some crude methods were tried to prevent the disease, but it was not until much later, the late 1700s, when methods closer to today's vaccines and vaccinations began to evolve and started to solve problems associated with disease.

Vaccination, according to *Merriam-Webster*, is "the introduction into humans or domestic animals of microorganisms that have previously been treated to make them harmless for the purpose of inducing the development of immunity." This is similar to what British doctor Edward Jenner did in 1796 when he devised a system of transferring live cowpox virus into a person's arm in order to protect them from developing smallpox. Jenner's technique worked. A young boy was seemingly protected from smallpox.

Interestingly, not everyone at the time was convinced in this medical breakthrough. People questioned it, fought against it, and used the social media of the time, the newspapers, to spread their fury against the early vaccines and vaccinations. They also joined anti-vaccination associations. An American Anti-Vaccination Society formed in 1879 questioned the motives of health officials, politicians, and pharmaceutical companies, claiming their motives were based on financial gain instead of health outcomes. Knowledge and techniques in medicine continued to improve, and by the 20th century the number of vaccines in use had increased. When Jonas Salk invented the polio vaccine, he became a hero. By 1971, the MMR vaccine, for measles, mumps, and rubella, had arrived. As time marched along, vaccine science produced more treatments, and eventually the vaccines for COVID-19, developed in record time, worked to tackle the novel virus that had caused a modern pandemic.

Even though the World Health Organization (WHO) says that "immunization is one of modern medicine's greatest success stories" and that it "prevents deaths every year in all age groups from diseases like diphtheria, tetanus, pertussis (whooping cough), influenza and measles," there are individuals and groups who vehemently argue against its practice. It happened back in Edward Jenner's time, and it continues today with the anti-vaxx movement. Researchers know that "just 12 people are responsible for the bulk of the misleading claims and outright lies about COVID-19 vaccines that proliferate on Facebook, Instagram and Twitter."[1]

Misinformation strewn about on social media isn't the only thing causing vaccine hesitancy. Political affiliation is a big cause. A Gallup survey released in 2021 confirmed that political affiliation is a factor in COVID-19 vaccine hesitancy, far surpassing earlier factors such as race and ethnicity. At the time of the survey 92% of Democrats, 68% of Independents, and only 56% of Republicans had been vaccinated.[2]

This polarization is more than a social or political issue: it's a public health issue. Vaccines will be a necessity in the future.

Some scientists and medical experts argue that now is the time to prepare for the next pandemic. Experts are searching for the next potential source of zoonotic disease, and others maintain that humans must curtail climate change and its associated ecological effects to prevent upcoming pandemics. And almost everyone agrees that global cooperation is a fundamental necessity for worldwide positive health outcomes.

Opposing Viewpoints: Vaccines offers diverse perspectives on a topic that many assumed was not at all polarizing. In chapters titled "How Do Vaccines Impact Public and Private Health?"; "Has Media Affected the Acceptance of Vaccines?"; "Does Politics Alter the Perception of Vaccines in Society?"; and "What Is the Future for Vaccines?" viewpoint authors explore this very timely debate.

Notes

1. Shannon Bond, "Just 12 People Are Behind Most Vaccine Hoaxes On Social Media, Research Shows," NPR, May 14, 2021.
2. William A. Galston, "For COVID-19 Vaccinations, Party Affiliation Matters More Than Race and Ethnicity," Brookings, October 1, 2021.

OPPOSING VIEWPOINTS® SERIES

Chapter 1

How Do Vaccines Impact Public and Private Health?

Chapter Preface

Vaccines, it appears, have been controversial since their inception. Even with the advancement of medicine and treatments available today, a great many people distrust the medical establishment. It is understandable that back in the late 1790s when the smallpox vaccination was first developed, people mistrusted the practice. However, there also have been times when people, especially parents, trusted in science and rushed to get themselves and their children vaccinated.

The viewpoints in the following chapter reflect varying stances on this hotly debated topic. Many use information and knowledge gained from the COVID-19 pandemic. Are vaccines safe? Do they protect against disease? Do the potential negative side effects outweigh the benefits? Some medical experts have maintained that immunity acquired from having COVID-19 is better than immunity from the COVID vaccine. On the surface, this appears to be indicated by solid statistics. But if true then why aren't more health officials agreeing? Could politics be interfering? Is it possible that the complexity of the human immune system proves that evolution has provided humans with a superior system of fighting disease to vaccine-induced immunity?

Included in the safety issues surrounding vaccines is the reporting of incidents of possible negative events. Of course, no medical treatment is totally without possible side effects. In a very different America in the 1950s, parents eagerly volunteered their children for vaccination testing in the fight against polio. This was a time when trust in science, medicine, and government was commonplace. Reading and contemplating the viewpoints in this chapter will provide insight into the issue of how vaccines impact public and private health.

Viewpoint 1

> *"It is very clear that vaccination against COVID-19 isn't as harmless as pharmaceuticals, mainstream media, academia, health authorities and the medical community have been saying."*

Natural Immunity Is a Better Choice Against COVID-19 Infection

Marc Girardot

In the following viewpoint Marc Girardot makes an argument for the natural immunity a body possesses after being infected and recovered from COVID-19 as opposed to relying on vaccine-induced immunity proposed by many health initiatives. Girardot argues that a body's natural immunity is a system that was perfected during human evolution and thereby a complicated, but robust natural survival mechanism. He further questions the validity of whether survivors of COVID-19 should elect to be vaccinated against the disease or its variants. Marc Girardot's expertise lies in business and economics ,with training and experience in the scientific method, biotech, and energy.

As you read, consider the following questions:

1. According to the author, is the COVID-19 vaccine causing adverse effects?

"Best of 2021: Natural Immunity vs Covid-19 Vaccine-Induced Immunity—Marc Girardot of PANDA," by Marc Girardot, Biznews, December 16, 2021. Reprinted by permission. https://www.biznews.com/undictated/2021/12/16/best-2021-immunity-covid-19-vaccine.

2. As reported by the viewpoint, which diseases did people have immunity against even after years of lessening body responses?
3. Does the author denigrate all vaccines?

A British friend, recovered from COVID, decided to get vaccinated despite being naturally immune. This is the email he recently sent me:

> Marc I suffered a mild stroke on Wednesday 8 days after taking the Astrazeneca 2nd dose. Since I am a marathon runner I am a very "rare case". I don't smoke, have high blood pressure, high cholesterol, family history or come into any of the risk categories for blood clots…
>
> You did warn me against taking the second dose and I wished I'd heeded your advice. I've taken a totally unnecessary risk with my life and I bitterly regret doing it.

Contrary to most, Tony was informed; he had been told about the power of natural immunity, about the long—if not lifelong—duration of immunity, of the risk inherent to any medical procedure (yes, vaccination is a medical procedure!), as well as of the rising levels of adverse events. He admitted he hadn't imagined it could happen to him…

Though it is hard to assess precisely the actual severity and breadth of vaccine-related adverse events, it is very clear that vaccination against COVID-19 isn't as harmless as pharmaceuticals, mainstream media, academia, health authorities and the medical community have been saying. And, in contrast to high risk individuals who are still susceptible, recovered people have no real benefit to balance the additional risks of vaccination.

For over a year, mainstream media, health authorities as well as many "experts" have been downplaying the power of the immune system, dismissing natural immunity and proclaiming that immunity to COVID-19 was short-lived. Simultaneously, vaccines have been portrayed as the silver bullet to this crisis, an incidental procedure with no risk whatsoever. The data shows a different picture and many are coming forward, to challenge the official narrative. We will demonstrate that this is a fallacy.

The human immune system is one of the most sophisticated achievements of evolution. The survival of our species has depended on it for millenia. And today, we are still very much relying on it. For the record, 99% of people infected with SARS-CoV-2 recover without treatment. Only 1% of SARS-CoV-2 patients, who did not receive early home-based treatment, end up hospitalised. In other words, the immune system overwhelmingly protects. Even vaccines depend entirely on the immune system: vaccines essentially teach our immune systems what viral markers to be prepared for, they are not cures per se. Without a functional immune system, there can be no effective vaccine.

On the Waning Immunity Fallacy

Once recovered, the immune response recedes, notably via a decrease in antibodies. It is not only natural; it is indispensable to restore the body to a normal balanced state. Just as a permanent state of fever would be harmful, a high number of targetless antibodies or T-cells constantly circulating throughout the body could create serious complications such as autoimmune diseases. Taking an evolutionary perspective, only those whose antibody and T-cells count waned post-infection survived. So, a dropping number of antibodies and T-cells is reassuring, even healthy.

But this decrease in T-cells and antibodies doesn't mean at all that immunity is gone. It means the immune system has adapted to the new situation, and is now just on sentinel mode: Memory B- and T-cells, circulating in the blood and resident in tissues, act as vigilant and effective sentinels for decades:

- survivors of the Spanish Flu epidemic were tested for their immunity to the 1918 influenza virus 90 years after, and still demonstrated immunity;
- people recovered from the 2003 SARS infection demonstrated robust T-cell responses seventeen years later;

- the wide-spread prevalence of high cross-immunity—gained from past common cold infections—further demonstrates the resilience of natural immunity for coronaviruses.

Indeed, all recent studies show the specific anti-SARS-CoV-2 immunity remains effective—possibly for a lifetime. Our immune system is a modular platform, it can combine in an infinite number of ways to address a multitude of threats in a variety of contexts. As such, it is neutral to the viral threats it faces. In other words, there is absolutely no reason to believe that those recovered from COVID-19 would lose their immunity over the years, or even the decades to come.

On the Reinfection Fallacy

You might have also heard of people becoming reinfected by SARS-CoV-2. Indeed, immunity, natural or vaccine-induced, isn't the impenetrable shield described by many. Essentially harmless and asymptomatic reinfections do take place. That is, in fact, the very mechanism by which adaptive immunity is triggered.

However, symptomatic reinfections are very rare. Like an army which adapts its response to the size and the progression of its enemy forces, adaptive immunity provides a specific, rapid and resource-optimised response. As such, reinfections are mostly asymptomatic and recovered patients are protected from severe disease.

In fact, innocuous reinfections can play a positive public health role as continuous immune updates of the population. They can help a seamless and progressive adaptation to emerging new variants and strains. And indeed a recent study showed that couples with children were more frequently asymptomatic than couples without, most likely because children acted as natural and harmless immunisation vehicles. The likely reason high density countries all have very low death tolls is that they have asymptomatic reinfections that regularly and widely update the immunity of the population.

On the Variant Fallacy

As demonstrated by the low numbers of reinfections mentioned above, but also by multiple studies, so far variants have not escaped acquired immunity. Just as Americans can speak and interact seamlessly in England, unhindered by a few word variants, natural or vaccine-induced immunity is unhindered by variants, possibly more so than vaccine-induced immunity. There is ample evidence of the sophistication and breadth of the human immune system, and it is clear that its arsenal cannot be evaded by a few minor changes in the genes of the virus.

Across the world (countries: Canada, Ecuador, Gabon, Germany, India, Singapore, Sweden, UK, USA, Tanzania, Zambia), multiple studies demonstrate high-levels of pre-existing cross-reactive T-cells and antibodies to SARS-CoV-2. In other words, many were already largely immune via other coronaviruses. This is the likely explanation for the unexpectedly high level of asymptomatics during the pandemic. More importantly, this demonstrates that even with large genetic differences, prior immunity to related coronaviruses is sufficient to avoid severe Covid. Therefore, it is quite evident [that] variants are not a concern for the general population who have already recovered.

On the Vaccine Better-than-the-Natural-Immunity Fallacy

You might have heard people stating that vaccines provide better protection than natural immunity. That's an interesting way of bending reality. How can a vaccine be more effective at immunisation than the disease it is trying to mimic?

Theoretically, there are several reasons explaining why natural immunity is better than vaccine-induced immunity:

- Fewer immune targets: mRNA/DNA vaccines present only a fraction of the virus genetic code (5-10%). For example, they don't utilise ORF1 highly immunogenic epitopes. Therefore, the immune system will recruit a smaller number of T-cells tapping into a narrower repertoire, consequently with a less effective response. The logic: Imagine you lose a number of key players for a football tournament—you might still win, but it will be harder.

- Longer immune trigger time: The smaller number of epitope targets also means that the alarm to the immune system will be delayed. This is a key driver of success in the COVID-19 battle. The wider the target repertoire, the faster the encounter between dendritic cells and identifiable antigens. The logic: Like a party you go to, you can start partying much faster when you have ten friends there than when you have only one. They are just easier to find.
- Inappropriate delivery location: The intramuscular delivery of current vaccines unfortunately doesn't mimic viral penetration and propagation at all. Coronaviruses don't enter the body via muscles. They do so via the respiratory tract, often infecting cell to cell. Contrary to muscle-delivered vaccines, natural immunity places a strong sentinel force of memory resident cells at the portals of entry and shuts the body entrance to the virus preemptively. From an evolutionary standpoint, this makes perfect sense. The logic: It's much easier to stop an army coming through a narrow gorge than on the beaches of Normandy.

Recent research confirms this logic. One comparative study in Israel found the protection from severe disease to be 96.4% for COVID-19 recovered individuals but 94.4% for vaccinated ones, and concluded "Our results question the need to vaccinate previously-infected individuals." Another reference comparative study by a team at New York University highlighted a faster, wider and more impactful humoral and cytotoxic reaction in recovered immunity versus vaccine-induced.

There is ample evidence that vaccinating people recovered from COVID doesn't bring any benefit. It quite possibly does the opposite, because of the risk of building tolerance to elements of the virus translating into reduced immune potency.

On the Vaccine Innocuity Fallacy

Without denigrating the incredible contribution of vaccines to modern medicine and public health, one needs to acknowledge that vaccines are a medical procedure. As such, vaccines should never be considered lightly. They are neither neutral, nor trivial, all the more so when they are injected into billions of people.

In their very nature, vaccines tinker with the sophisticated balance of one's immune system. That in itself demands respecting rigid safety protocols. Though we have made considerable progress in our understanding of immunology, we are still very far from understanding its intricacies and subtleties, especially when it comes to novel mRNA and DNA technologies.

Because of the risk of anaphylactic shock, auto-immune diseases, unforeseen interactions, design flaws, deficient quality protocols, over-dosage, and so on—vaccines have traditionally been strictly regulated.

History teaches us to be watchful with vaccines, from the botched inactivation of polio vaccines that ended infecting 40,000 kids with polio in 1955, to the 1976 swine flu vaccine which caused 450 to develop Guillain-Barré syndrome, to the more recent vaccine-induced outbreak of polio in Sudan. The recent rejection by Brazilian health authorities of the Barhat's Covaxin is a clear reminder of how rigorous and independent our health authorities need to be if vaccines are to promote, not hinder, public health.

After 6 months of vaccination and a year of research, a number of red signals should be alerting the would-be vaccinated and health authorities:

1. Wandering nanoparticles: The lipid nanoparticles, the carriers of the mRNA, were supposed to remain in the muscle, but ended up broadly distributed throughout the body, notably in the ovaries, the liver and possibly the bone marrow.
2. Anaphylactic PEG: A number of concerns had been raised regarding the novel use of PEG adjuvant. Notably, prior

research had raised the risk of cardiac anaphylaxis at second injection.

3. Sensitive locations: ACE-2 receptors susceptible to binding to the spike protein are highly expressed in the endothelial cells of highly sensitive areas, such as the brain, the heart, the lungs, the liver and both male and female reproductive systems.
4. Toxic circulating spikes: The spike proteins induced by mRNA/DNA vaccines have been shown to be pathogenic, and highly inflammatory, notably because of the similarity of a spike sequence to that of Staphylococcal Enterotoxin B. It has also been found to be directly causing blood clots through platelet activation. One researcher said, "Our findings show that the SARS-CoV-2 spike protein causes lung injury even without the presence of an intact virus."
5. BBB disruption: A recent study highlights the risk of disruption of the blood-brain barrier, a fundamental filter mechanism to protect the brain. The spike protein has also been found to cross the BBB and create inflammation in the brain.
6. High adverse events: Even though most likely under-reported, the overall number of serious adverse events versus other traditional vaccines remains very high. The 6,000+ deaths seen [in the US] in six months exceed all the vaccine-related deaths in 30 years. This is quite disquieting, and tends to confirm the aforementioned alarms.
7. Children more at risk: The COVID-19 vaccines seem to be more harmful to children and teens, notably with a growing number of myocarditis events. The fact that vaccine doses are not adjusted for body weight is notably a cause for concern given the discovery of circulating nanoparticles and spike toxicity.

These are essentially just the short-term effects of these novel vaccines. There is no long-term clinical data regarding the implications of these vaccines, notably regarding autoreactive antibodies (antibodies that target one's own body creating autoimmune diseases).

To conclude, we question why anyone healthy and recovered from COVID-19 would want or be advised to take any risk—even the most remote—in getting vaccinated given that:

- those who have recovered from COVID-19 enjoy robust immunity;
- natural immunity duration is decades-long, probably lifelong;
- natural immunity effectiveness is better than vaccine-induced;
- variants are not an immunological concern, presenting no risk of immune escape;
- vaccines are medical interventions which should never be taken lightly, especially when still experimental;
- there is no benefit for COVID-19 recovered; and
- COVID-19 vaccines are obviously not as safe as stated initially by the manufacturers.

Viewpoint 2

> *"All COVID-19 vaccines approved by WHO for emergency use listing have been through randomized clinical trials to test their quality, safety and efficacy."*

Vaccines Are Safe and Reliable

World Health Organization

In the following viewpoint the World Health Organization outlines the effectiveness of the COVID-19 vaccine and the reasons for its use as a public health measure. The WHO explains the role of efficacy and effectiveness of vaccines and the possible reasons of breakthrough infections. Simple precautions against infection are outlined in the viewpoint as well as cautionary notes about virus variants. The World Health Organization is a specialized unit of the United Nations and is responsible for overseeing international public health issues.

As you read, consider the following questions:

1. What is a vaccine's efficacy as outlined in the viewpoint article?
2. As reported by WHO, how fast does an inoculated person attain protection from a vaccine?
3. According to the viewpoint, what does the COVID-19 vaccination protect against?

Reproduced from World Health Organization, "Vaccine Efficacy, Effectiveness and Protection," July 14, 2021. Reprinted by permission.

This article is part of a series of explainers on vaccine development and distribution. Learn more about vaccines—from how they work and how they're made to ensuring safety and equitable access—in WHO's Vaccines Explained series.

COVID-19 vaccines have proven to be safe, effective and life-saving. Like all vaccines, they do not fully protect everyone who is vaccinated, and we do not yet know how well they can prevent people from transmitting the virus to others. So as well as getting vaccinated, we must also continue with other measures to fight the pandemic.

Vaccine Efficacy and Effectiveness

All COVID-19 vaccines approved by WHO for emergency use listing have been through randomized clinical trials to test their quality, safety and efficacy. To be approved, vaccines are required to have a high efficacy rate of 50% or above. After approval, they continue to be monitored for ongoing safety and effectiveness. But what is the difference between efficacy and effectiveness?

A vaccine's efficacy is measured in a controlled clinical trial and is based on how many people who got vaccinated developed the "outcome of interest" (usually disease) compared with how many people who got the placebo (dummy vaccine) developed the same outcome. Once the study is complete, the numbers of sick people in each group are compared, in order to calculate the relative risk of getting sick depending on whether or not the subjects received the vaccine. From this we get the efficacy—a measure of how much the vaccine lowered the risk of getting sick. If a vaccine has high efficacy, a lot fewer people in the group who received the vaccine got sick than the people in the group who received the placebo.

So, for example, let's imagine a vaccine with a proven efficacy of 80%. This means that—out of the people in the clinical trial—those who received the vaccine were at a 80% lower risk of developing disease than the group who received the placebo. This is calculated by comparing the number of cases of disease in the vaccinated group versus the placebo group. An efficacy of 80% does not mean that 20% of the vaccinated group will become ill.

Vaccine effectiveness is a measure of how well vaccines work in the real world. Clinical trials include a wide range of people—a broad age range, both sexes, different ethnicities and those with known medical conditions—but they cannot be a perfect representation of the whole population. The efficacy seen in clinical trials applies to specific outcomes in a clinical trial . Effectiveness is measured by observing how well the vaccines work to protect communities as a whole. Effectiveness in the real world can differ from the efficacy measured in a trial, because we can't predict exactly how effective

Is Natural Immunity Effective Against Viruses?

Dr. Marty Makary, a professor at John Hopkins School of Medicine, during an appearance on The Vince Coglianese Show, said individuals formerly infected with COVID-19 are seven times more likely than vaccinated people to fight off the virus.

"It appears that natural immunity is better against the Delta variant. When you get infected with COVID, your body's immune system develops antibodies to the entire surface of the virus," Makary said. "Not just the slight protein that the vaccines gives you, but the entire surface. And so you get a more diverse antibody portfolio in your system."

Makary said data from Israel revealed that natural immunity appears to be 6.7x more effective than being vaccinated when it comes to fighting off COVID-19.

"One of the great failures of our medical leadership has been ignoring the half of America with natural immunity, which is the half of non-vaccinated folks."

vaccination will be for a much bigger and more variable population getting vaccinated in more real life conditions.

Vaccine Protection and Timing

Vaccines offer strong protection, but that protection takes time to build. People must take all the required doses of a vaccine to build full immunity. For two-dose vaccines, vaccines only give partial protection after the first dose, and the second dose increases that protection. It takes time before protection reaches its maximum level a few weeks after the second dose. For a one-dose vaccine, people will have built maximum immunity against COVID-19 a few weeks after getting vaccinated.

> Host Vince Coglianese said that the government likely does not share this data because "they're scared that people are going to try and take the risk."
>
> Makary has still encouraged those who are not vaccinated and not immune to get the vaccine.
>
> Studies conducted by researchers from the Washington University School of Medicine in St. Louis found that cells in the bone marrow of those who recovered from COVID a year earlier had a memory of the virus. Another study showed that the cells continue to mature 12 months after the individual contracted the virus.
>
> Dr. William Hanage, an associate professor of epidemiology at Harvard's T.H. Chan School of Public Health, said that it is "impossible" to know whether the COVID vaccine or natural immunity is more protective against the virus due to the lack of knowledge regarding the level of protection natural immunity gives a person over time. Reinfection occurs in about 10% of people after having contracted the virus as a result of a decrease in immunity over time.
>
> **"Dr. Makary Says Natural Immunity Is More Effective than Vaccine Immunity," by Nicole Silverio, The Daily Caller, August 5, 2021.**

Vaccine Protection and Infection

Vaccines can stop most people from getting sick with COVID-19, but not everyone.

Even after someone takes all of the recommended doses and waits a few weeks for immunity to build up, there is still a chance that they can get infected. Vaccines do not provide full (100%) protection, so "breakthrough infections"—where people get the virus, despite having been fully vaccinated—will occur.

If vaccinated people do get sick, they are likely to have milder symptoms, in general It is very rare for someone vaccinated to experience severe illness or die.

Vaccine Protection and Transmission

COVID-19 vaccines are crucial tools in the pandemic response and protect against severe disease and death. Vaccines provide at least some protection from infection and transmission, but not as much as the protection they provide against serious illness and death. More evidence is needed to determine exactly how well they stop infection and transmission.

After being vaccinated, individuals should continue taking simple precautions, such as physical distancing, wearing a mask, keeping rooms well ventilated, avoiding crowds, cleaning hands, and coughing into a bent elbow or tissue. Get tested if you are sick, even if you've been vaccinated. Check local advice where you live and work. Do it all!

Vaccine Protection and Variants

When cases increase and transmission accelerates, it's more likely that new dangerous and more transmissible variants emerge, which can spread more easily or cause more severe illness.

Based on what we know so far, vaccines are proving effective against existing variants, especially at preventing severe disease, hospitalization and death. However, some variants are having a slight impact on the ability of vaccines to guard against mild disease and infection.

Vaccines are likely staying effective against variants because of the broad immune response they cause, which means that virus changes or mutations are unlikely to make vaccines completely ineffective.

WHO continues to constantly review the evidence and will update its guidance as we find out more. For the latest updates on what we know about the COVID-19 variants, read our latest weekly epidemiological updates and our explainer on "the effects of virus variants on COVID-19 vaccines."

One of the best ways of guarding against new variants is to continue applying tried-and-tested public health measures and rolling out vaccines. All COVID-19 vaccines approved for emergency use listing by WHO have been thoroughly tested and proven to provide a high degree of protection against serious illness and death. As stronger virus variants emerge, it's important to take your vaccine when it's your turn.

Viewpoint 3

> "...*in 1955, many Americans had an especially deep respect for science.*"

In the Past, People Eagerly Sought the Protection of Vaccines

Barbara Pfeffer Billauer

In the following viewpoint Barbara Pfeffer Billauer maintains that at one time Americans fully embraced and respected the scientific development of vaccines. Billauer contends that even though adverse reactions happened, people eagerly sought out vaccines and enrolled their children in vaccine testing programs. Billauer analyzes the differences between then and now and proposes different reasons why vaccines are so mistrusted by many people today. Barbara Pfeffer Billauer is a professor of law and bioethics and a professor of research at the Institute of World Politics in Washington, DC.

As you read, consider the following questions:

1. As stated by the viewpoint, when did Americans have a respect for science?
2. According to the author, what are two reasons why people mistrust vaccinations?
3. At the peak of their disease state, which killed more people, COVID-19 or polio?

"Once There Was a Time, When Vaccine Uptake Was Robust," by Barbara Pfeffer Billauer, The American Council on Science and Health, September 29, 2021. Reprinted by permission. https://www.acsh.org/news/2021/09/29/once-there-was-time-when-vaccine-uptake-was-robust-15837#_msocom_2

The year was 1947—the last smallpox invasion in America. Ground zero: New York City. The carrier: an ex-pat named Eugene LeBar, who had arrived from Mexico on March 1. By the time his diagnosis was confirmed, more than a month later, he had likely exposed thousands of New Yorkers. Even before arriving in New York, LeBar had traveled through seven major American population centers, exposing probably hundreds more.

Smallpox in the Big Apple

Once the diagnosis was confirmed, New York City's Mayor, William O'Dwyer, reacted quickly, issuing an appeal for universal vaccination. His constituents responded immediately. In the space of two weeks, five million people were vaccinated, two and a half million in the first week alone. In less than a month, more than 84% of the City's population of 7,500,000 were vaccinated. There were no lawsuits, no riots, no opposition. People quietly and courteously lined up to be vaccinated. A month later, the epidemic was declared over.

Maybe the Jacobson case from Massachusetts forty years prior had primed the populace. Maybe people were war-weary. Maybe the health commissioner, Dr. Israel Weinstein, and his daily radio programs, were better at risk-communication than we are now. Maybe people were freaked out. Maybe there were no organized anti-vax groups spouting propaganda or groups urging personal choice, stoking the populace?

It wasn't because the vaccine was readily available. At the time the campaign was announced, there were 250,000 doses on hand. O'Dwyer pressured vaccine manufacturers to step-up-to-the plate and expedite vaccine production. More than 1,000 physicians, 242 clerks, and 3,000 civilian volunteers did the vaccinating, while NYC's finest supervised the long lines snaking around vaccine centers. All the while, Dr. Weinstein calmly countered the hysterical media in his daily radio broadcasts [BB2].

It wasn't because the smallpox vaccine was especially safe. That vaccine is one of the most dangerous vaccines made. Because of the manner of its formulation and its long history of tetanus-causing contamination, people were genuinely and validly frightened [1]. When 500,000 smallpox vaccines were allocated to the CDC in 2003 for first responders in the wake of Saddam's alleged production of a smallpox bioweapon, the [BB3] uptake was minimal; only 38,000 volunteered in the first eight months. Fear of the vaccine coupled with the low likelihood that such a weapon would ever materialize drove that wave of vaccine refusal. A New England Journal of Medicine article confirmed the low risk-benefit ratio of vaccinating the general public from a terrorist attack.

Yet, the reaction after the smallpox virus actually made landfall in New York in 1947 was swift, silent, and orderly. Vaccine uptake was high enough to provide herd immunity.

Smallpox Vaccine Fallout

By the time the epidemic was declared over

- Twelve people had contracted the disease; two had died. The case fatality was 16%, half the conventionally given number.
- Three people died of the vaccine; three more died from direct vaccine-related complications, for a total of six vaccine deaths. Another six died of probable vaccine-related encephalitis. No one cried foul. No one sued (at least to the best of my knowledge).

Polio

There was a similar experience with the polio vaccines, both Salk and Sabin. Here, too, the uptake was eager and accepted. Here, too, the vaccines were not completely benign. Here, too, there were instances of contamination. Yet, even at the experimental states, people rushed to have their children inoculated:

> In 1954 … frantic American parents—looking for anything that could beat back the horror of polio—offered up more than 1.8 million children to serve as test subjects. They included 600,000 kids who would be injected with either a new polio

> vaccine or a placebo.... 443,000 children received at least one polio inoculation, while more than 210,000 received a placebo....

There was no vaccine resistance. There were no concerns about autism. But then, there was no Andrew Wakefield spewing false associations of the vaccine with autism. Nor was there RFK Jr. spouting that vaccines do not prevent disease.

So, What's the Difference Between Then and Now?

"One reason, historians say, is that in 1955, many Americans had an especially deep respect for science." [NPR, 2021]

One reason might have been greater forthcomingness and honesty. Even mishaps in vaccine manufacturing did not diminish the parent's trust in the vaccine, the program, or the leaders of the vaccination program. That trust must have been huge:

In 1955, 200,000 children received a defective polio vaccine when live virus was mistakenly used instead of the killed virus specified. Forty thousand got polio; 200 were left with paralysis; ten died. Nevertheless, even afterward, mothers and fathers jumped right back in, once again signing permission slips and lining their kids up to get their polio shot.

One reason might have been rank terror. Smallpox conjured horrors of a physically disgusting disease. And while American epidemics since the turn of the last century were far less lethal than previously, the mythic mantra of a 30% smallpox case-fatality rate remains embedded in the American medical literature [2]. Polio left some of its survivors paralyzed or disabled. The grossly unattractive physical remnants of both diseases were obvious. People did what they could to avoid them—lockdowns were voluntarily implemented:

"As [polio] outbreaks popped up across the country in the hot summer months, people were terrified and voluntarily isolated...." "Back then, it affected business and travel," says Stacey D. Stewart, current president and CEO of the March of Dimes. "People didn't know how the virus was transmitted. They lived in a state of fear.

Pools were closed. Businesses were affected because people didn't want to be out in public."

Perhaps it's because the anti-vaxxers have taken control of the public relations campaign. Their message: fear the vaccine; don't fear vaccine-preventable diseases, be they COVID or measles, they aren't dangerous, and above all, don't trust the evil pharmaceutical industry or the duplicitous government.

Perhaps, there is a false sense of invulnerability, an arrogant assumption of invincibility, or a legitimate but greater dependence on economic grease for survival compared to 75 years ago. In the middle of the last century, polio disabled an average of 35,000 people a year in the U.S., mostly children. In 1952, the peak year, 3000 children died. So far, COVID has claimed the lives of 680,000 Americans. This chilling statistic doesn't seem to move either the rank anti-vaxxers or their deceptively disarming allies who extoll individual freedom as a basis to resist public health measures and vaccine mandates, all the while proclaiming their support of vaccination.

Perhaps today, legitimately, people are more mistrusting of government. The organized anti-vax movement seems to have found rich (unwitting) allies, augmenting their coffers, power, and reach. Destabilizing groups falsely urge the assumption of autonomy, personal control, and unlimited personal freedom to reject vaccines even when the health of others is at stake. Others, seemingly pro-vaccines, reject governmental intercession as a matter of principle, even when vaccine mandates may be our only alternative.

Most (maybe all) public health lawyers, myself included, would prefer that vaccine mandates or compelled vaccination would never be needed. In our past, that was sometimes the case, but maybe today, we need more public health tools in our arsenal.

Ideologies can be noble. But survival is necessary. Sometimes we must sacrifice our lives for our beliefs. But sometimes, we must sacrifice our beliefs to live, to fight again another day. The crux of wisdom is determining which is time is now. It used to be that science helped answer the questions. No longer, it seems.

Notes

1. Michael Willrich, Pox (2011)
2. Harrison's Textbook of Internal Medicine in 1970 noted the case-fatality of smallpox was 20%

Additional Sources: Weapons of Mass Hysteria, Faulty Biothreat Predictions, and Their Impact on National (In)Security: A Case-Study of Smallpox, Health Matrix Journal of Law-Medicine (2017)

Viewpoint 4

> *"...in truth, few things meet the definition of 'harmless.' Even everyday activities contain hidden dangers."*

Do Benefits of Vaccines Outweigh the Risks?

Children's Hospital of Philadelphia

In the following viewpoint Children's Hospital of Philadelphia (CHOP) analyzes whether vaccines are truly safe. CHOP details three different vaccines and analyzes the diseases that are prevented because of the vaccines. CHOP also present statistics that illuminate why the benefits of vaccines outweigh the risks, and the systems used to detect potential vaccine problems. Children's Hospital of Philadelphia is an elite pediatric hospital.

As you read, consider the following questions:

1. What is an example of an everyday situation causing death, as reported by this viewpoint?
2. Which country outlawed the pertussis vaccine?
3. Which two systems monitor vaccine safety?

The first definition of the word safe is "harmless." This definition would imply that any negative consequence of a vaccine would make the vaccine unsafe. Using this definition, no vaccine

"Vaccine Safety: Are Vaccines Safe?" Children's Hospital of Philadelphia. Vaccine Education Center (Vaccine.chop.edu May19, 2020 version). Reprinted by permission.

is 100 percent safe. Almost all vaccines can cause pain, redness or tenderness at the site of injection. And some vaccines cause more severe side effects. For example, the original pertussis (whooping cough) vaccine could cause persistent, inconsolable crying, high fever or seizures associated with fever. Although none of these severe symptoms resulted in permanent damage, they could be quite frightening to parents.

But, in truth, few things meet the definition of "harmless." Even everyday activities contain hidden dangers. For example, every year in the United States, about 350 people are killed in bath- or shower-related accidents, about 5,000 people are killed when food lodges in their windpipe, and about 50 people are struck and killed by lightning. However, few of us consider taking a bath, eating solid food or walking outside on a rainy day as unsafe activities. We just figure that the benefits of the activity outweigh the risks.

The second definition of the word safe is "having been preserved from a real danger." Using this definition, the danger (the disease) must be significantly greater than the means of protecting against the danger (the vaccine). Or, said another way, a vaccine's benefits must clearly and definitively outweigh its risks.

To better understand the definition of the word safe when applied to vaccines, let's examine a few different vaccines and the diseases they prevent.

Is the Hepatitis B Vaccine Safe?

The hepatitis B vaccine has few side effects. However, one side effect is serious. About 1 of every 1 million doses of hepatitis B vaccine is complicated by a severe allergic reaction, called anaphylaxis. The symptoms of anaphylaxis are hives, difficulty breathing and a drop in blood pressure. Although no one has ever died because of the hepatitis B vaccine, the symptoms of anaphylaxis caused by the vaccine can be quite frightening.

On the other hand, every year about 1,700 people die in the United States soon after being infected with hepatitis B virus. And, millions of people throughout the world live with chronic hepatitis B infection. Between 1 and 2 million of these people live in the United States. Up to 1 in 4 chronically infected people will suffer severe liver damage (called cirrhosis) or liver cancer caused by hepatitis B virus. People are much more likely to develop these severe, and often fatal, consequences of hepatitis B virus infection if they get infected when they are very young children. For this reason, the hepatitis B vaccine is recommended for newborns.

Some parents wonder whether it is necessary to give the hepatitis B virus vaccine to newborns. They ask: "How is a baby going to catch hepatitis B?" But, before the hepatitis B virus vaccine, every year in the United States about 18,000 children less than 10 years of age caught hepatitis B virus from someone other than their mother. Some children caught it from another family member, and some children caught it from someone outside the home who came into contact with the baby.

Although about 1 to 2 million people in the United States are infected with hepatitis B virus, many of these are "silent infections," meaning without obvious symptoms. As a result, many people who are infected with hepatitis B virus don't know that they have it. So it can be hard to tell from whom you could catch hepatitis B virus.

Worse yet, many people don't realize that you can catch hepatitis B virus after coming into contact with very small quantities of blood—small enough that they are not visible to the naked eye. This means that someone can be infected through relatively casual contact with someone who is infected, such as sharing washcloths or toothbrushes. In fact, a milliliter of blood (about one-fifth of a teaspoon) from someone who is infected can contain as many as 1 billion infectious viruses.

Because the benefits of the hepatitis B vaccine clearly and definitively outweigh its risks, the hepatitis B vaccine is safe.

Was the Old Pertussis Vaccine Safe?

The old pertussis vaccine had far more risks than the hepatitis B vaccine. The old pertussis vaccine was called the "whole-cell" vaccine and had a high rate of severe side effects. Persistent, inconsolable crying occurred in 1 of every 100 doses, fever greater than 105 degrees Fahrenheit occurred in 1 of every 100 doses, and seizures with fever occurred in 1 of every 1,750 doses. Due to negative publicity related to this vaccine, its use decreased in many areas of the world.

For example, the Japanese Ministry of Health decided to stop using the pertussis vaccine in 1975. In the three years before the vaccine was discontinued, 400 cases of pertussis and 10 deaths from pertussis occurred in Japan. In 1979, four years after the pertussis vaccine was discontinued, 13,000 cases of pertussis and 41 deaths were reported. It should be noted that although the side effects of the pertussis vaccine were real, children didn't die from pertussis vaccine; however, they did die from pertussis infection. The Japanese Ministry of Health, realizing how costly their error had been, soon reinstituted use of pertussis vaccine.

The decisions in Japan proved that, despite the side effects, the benefits of the old pertussis vaccine clearly outweighed the risks.

Scientific progress eventually led to the creation of another version of the pertussis vaccine. Known as the "acellular" pertussis vaccine, it was more purified, so instead of containing about 3,000 immunogenic proteins, it only contained two to five proteins. The ("acellular") pertussis vaccine became available in the United States in 1996. Children who received this vaccine had a much lower risk of severe side effects than those who received the old "whole-cell" vaccine. Therefore, the new pertussis vaccine is safer than the old pertussis vaccine. But because the benefits of the old pertussis vaccine outweighed its risks, it too was safe.

Is the Pneumococcal Vaccine Safe?

The pneumococcal vaccine was licensed in the United States in 2000 and was recommended for use in all children less than 5 years of age. Some parents chose to take a "wait-and-see" attitude. They reasoned that because the problems with the rotavirus vaccine were not revealed until the vaccine was given to 1 million children, why not wait and see what happened after the pneumococcal vaccine was given to several million or more children.

However, the choice not to give the pneumococcal vaccine was not a risk-free choice. Before pneumococcal vaccine was first given to infants in 2000, every year in the United States about 700 children (less than 5 years old) got meningitis, 17,000 got bloodstream infections, 5 million children developed ear infections, and 200 died from pneumococcus. So the choice not to get a pneumococcal vaccine was a choice to risk the consequences of pneumococcal infection, which were occasionally fatal.

Parents should be reassured by two facts. First, the pneumococcal vaccine was tested in about 40,000 children before it was licensed for use. Second, the Haemophilus influenzae type b (Hib) vaccine is made in a manner almost identical to the pneumococcal vaccine (see How Are Vaccines Made?) and has been given safely to millions of children since 1990.

Detecting Rare Side Effects

The first rotavirus vaccine (RotaShield) is an example of how rare side effects can be detected quickly. The rotavirus vaccine was tested in about 11,000 children before it was submitted to the FDA for licensure. After the vaccine was licensed and recommended for use (see "Who licenses, recommends and requires vaccines?"), the vaccine was given to about 1 million children.

A system called the Vaccines Adverse Event Reporting System (VAERS) initially found about 15 cases of an intestinal blockage, called intussusception, soon after administration of the vaccine. This was worrisome enough to the Centers for Disease Control and Prevention (CDC) to cause them to temporarily suspend use of the rotavirus vaccine until it could be determined whether the vaccine did, in fact, cause intussusception. Their analysis showed that intussusception occurred in about 10 of every 100,000 children who received the vaccine. Because only 11,000 children were tested before the vaccine was licensed, it was really not possible to pick up such a rare side effect. The result of the rotavirus vaccine experience is that at least 60,000 children had to be tested before the next vaccine was licensed.

Several other systems of study to understand the rate of vaccine side effects, such as the Vaccine Safety Data Link (VSD), are also available. The VSD also allows one to determine the background rate of side effects, meaning the rate of adverse events in children who don't receive a vaccine. So, in many ways, systems like the Vaccine Safety Data Link are better than VAERS because they allow one to determine whether a particular vaccine is the cause of a rare side effect.

Viewpoint 5

"The data on natural immunity are now overwhelming"

Natural Immunity Is Underreported

Elizabeth Stauffer

In the following viewpoint Elizabeth Stauffer reports from the Johns Hopkins University School of Medicine that natural immunity acquired by having COVID-19 is proven to provide very good protection from the disease. Stauffer reports on findings, reiterated by Dr. Marty Makary, which demonstrate the proven protection inferred by contracting COVID-19, and in fact that herd immunity is being reached. Elizabeth Stauffer is a contract writer for The Western Journal and also for many conservative websites.

As you read, consider the following questions:

1. According to the viewpoint, is vaccine immunity or natural immunity better?
2. Is herd immunity occurring, according to experts quoted by the author?
3. Which US institutions have reported on the positive effects of natural immunity?

"Johns Hopkins Doc Says Vaccine Mandates 'Ruin Lives'—and Natural Immunity Is 27 Times Better Than Jab," by Elizabeth Stauffer, The Western Journal, January 28, 2022. Reprinted by permission.

The Biden administration's refusal to acknowledge the relevance of natural immunity in the fight against COVID-19 has become glaring.

The administration that constantly insists they are following the science is actually engaging in willful blindness.

Hell-bent on enforcing their COVID vaccine mandate, they deliberately ignore every scientific study that finds natural immunity to be superior to vaccine immunity.

Johns Hopkins University School of Medicine professor Dr. Marty Makary appeared as a guest on Thursday's edition of "Morning Wire," a podcast hosted by The Daily Wire.

"The data on natural immunity are now overwhelming," Makary told the Morning Wire. "It turns out the hypothesis that our public health leaders had that vaccinated immunity is better and stronger than natural immunity was wrong. They got it backwards. And now we've got data from Israel showing that natural immunity is 27 times more effective than vaccinated immunity. And that supports 15 other studies."

Despised by the left for his criticism of the vaccine mandate, Makary finds it bizarre that natural immunity is not seen as legitimate in the eyes of the U.S. government.

"It's ruining the lives of people who are getting fired," he said. "Nurses, who are heroes, are now getting laid off. Soldiers are getting dishonorably discharged. They've got immunity. It's just not the type that our public health officials have sanctioned."

"This is a failure of government, not a failure of science," he declared. "But how about some flexibility? How about recognizing natural immunity and allowing those who have circulating antibodies to get credit? That's how they do it in parts of Europe, and that's how they do it in Israel."

Makary said the recent drop-off in COVID cases can be attributed to both the tens of millions of Americans who have already had the virus and those who have been vaccinated.

The government refuses to acknowledge that the natural immunity acquired from having had COVID has played any role at all in moving us closer and faster to the desired goal of herd immunity. Makary is essentially saying natural immunity has played an enormous role.

This point is compelling and has been underreported.

"That decline [in new cases of COVID] is really natural immunity kicking in," Makary explained. "What we're seeing is that when a very few people in a population are susceptible, that is almost everybody has either had COVID or the vaccine. You do see this rapid decline. It's basically a part of herd immunity kicking in."

He believes "we're done with the surges. What we may see is bumping cases, seasonally, depending on pockets of the country where there's low immunity rates. And remember: breakthrough infections are real. They will happen, but they have downgraded COVID from a major public health threat to a mild, common, cold-like illness."

Makary feels that the vaccines are safe and that complications are "exceedingly rare." I know a few people who might disagree with that assessment.

At any rate, Makary told the Morning Wire, "When I talked to doctors nationwide, it's pretty clear that the vaccine-related complications are exceedingly rare and the vaccines we have are safer than any other vaccine we've ever had in the past. And I think if you if you're on the fence about getting vaccinated, you want to do it right now, like today, because we are getting to a point where it's so contagious, it's ripping through the population pretty quickly."

The consequences of the government's rejection of natural immunity as a valid reason to skip the vaccine have become apparent throughout the country, particularly in the health care industry and at all levels of law enforcement.

Democrats pushing Biden's misguided blanket vaccine mandate all parrot the same old tired line: "We follow the science." That's nonsense. It has nothing to do with science and everything to do with politics—the politics of power and control.

In a September Op-Ed published in The Washington Post, Makary wrote, "It's okay to have an incorrect scientific hypothesis. But when new data proves it wrong, you have to adapt. Unfortunately, many elected leaders and public health officials have held on far too long to the hypothesis that natural immunity offers unreliable protection against COVID-19—a contention that is being rapidly debunked by science."

Makary argued that over 15 studies have confirmed the power of natural immunity.

He cited the recent 700,000-person Israeli study which found that those who had recovered from COVID "were 27 times less likely to get a second symptomatic COVID infection than those who were vaccinated."

The results of the Israeli study, Makary wrote, confirmed the findings of a Cleveland Clinic study released in June. None of the health care workers who had previously contracted the virus were reinfected. The research team concluded that "individuals who have had SARS-CoV-2 infection are unlikely to benefit from COVID-19 vaccination."

And the Cleveland Clinic's results, he noted, affirmed the conclusions of a Washington University study conducted in May, which "found that even a mild COVID infection resulted in long-lasting immunity."

Maybe it's time for the Biden administration to take politics out of it and actually look at the science.

Viewpoint 6

> *"Evidence that shows COVID vaccination is primarily about individual health runs counter to the raison d'etre of the 'planners,' which is to exercise their plan over society."*

Vaccination Rates Are Not Linked to Lower COVID Rates

Jon Miltimore

In the following viewpoint Jon Miltimore argues that vaccines are a matter of personal health but not public health. Research cited by the author suggests that while the COVID vaccines offer individual protection, they do not contribute to herd immunity. Since they may not be improving public health, the author maintains, the argument for mandates is weak. Jon Miltimore is the Managing Editor of FEE. org. His writing/reporting has been the subject of articles in TIME magazine, The Wall Street Journal, CNN, Forbes, Fox News, and the Star Tribune.

As you read, consider the following questions:

1. What was interesting about Vermont's COVID case rate at the time of this viewpoint's original publication?

"Vaccination Rates Not Linked to Lower COVID Rates, Epidemiology Paper Finds," by Jon Miltimore, Foundation for Economic Education, October 15, 2021. https://fee.org/articles/vaccination-rates-not-linked-to-lower-covid-rates-epidemiology-paper-finds/. Licensed under CC BY-4.0 International.

2. Why does the author say that the vaccines help the health of the individual but not of the public?
3. Who is Ludwig von Mises, and why does the author use his observation to support his own argument?

On Friday, the San Francisco Chronicle published an article noting that California has some of the lowest COVID-19 case rates in the US, even though the Golden State's vaccination rate lags many states that are currently struggling with the delta variant.

"One clear example is the New England states of Vermont and Maine," the Chronicle reported. "Relatively shielded from the worst of the nation's previous surges, they have struggled against the delta variant, which has sent their case rates soaring."

In fact, Vermont has the highest vaccination rate in the country. Among those 65 years and older, 99.9 percent are fully vaccinated, and 74 percent of those 18-64 are fully vaccinated, according to data from the Mayo Clinic.

Yet, as the Chronicle points out, despite its high vaccination rate, Vermont recently set its single-day case record for the entire pandemic. And as of Oct. 1, Vermont's seven-day average case rate per 100k people was 30—triple that of the Bay Area.

What the Vaccines Do—and Don't Do

There is widespread agreement among scientists that COVID-19 vaccines are highly effective at reducing the risk of developing severe COVID symptoms, which can result in hospitalization and death.

Their effectiveness at reducing transmission of the virus, however, remains a subject of debate, particularly since the CDC released findings in July that show vaccinated individuals still contract the virus, transmit it, and carry just as many virus particles in their throat and nasal passages as unvaccinated individuals do when they contract the virus.

While scientists concede that the vaccines cannot stop transmission, many contend they still reduce transmission of the virus.

"We are confident vaccination against COVID-19 reduces the chances of transmitting the virus," Johns Hopkins epidemiologists M. Kate Grabowski and Justin Lessler argued in The Daily Beast.

Other scientists are less sure, and a new study suggests their skepticism may be warranted. The study, published last month in the European Journal of Epidemiology, a monthly peer-reviewed medical journal, examined 68 countries and 2,947 counties in the United States and concluded that higher vaccination rates are not associated with fewer COVID cases.

"At the country-level, there appears to be no discernable relationship between percentage of population fully vaccinated and new COVID-19 cases in the last 7 days," the researchers concluded. "In fact, the trend line suggests a marginally positive association such that countries with higher percentage of population fully vaccinated have higher COVID-19 cases per 1 million people." (emphasis added)

At the county level, the researchers said, there "also appears to be no significant signaling of COVID-19 cases decreasing with higher percentages of population fully vaccinated."

The findings do not suggest people shouldn't get vaccinated. Again, there's robust evidence showing vaccines reduce the risk of severe symptomatic COVID-19 reaction. What the research does suggest, however, is that vaccines are primarily a matter of personal health, not public health.

This is precisely what Dr. Jay Bhattacharya, a professor of medicine who studies epidemiology at Stanford, recently suggested. Bhattacharya noted that research indicates that the mRNA vaccines produced by Pfizer and Moderna offer abundant individual protection—Bhattacharya credits his own speedy recovery from COVID-19 to the vaccines—but don't contribute to herd immunity or improve public health.

Planned Chaos

The findings published in the European Journal of Epidemiology help explain why US states such as Vermont and Maine are suffering massive case outbreaks despite their high vaccination rates. (Public health experts also point out that California has much higher levels of natural immunity than its eastern counterparts, the Chronicle reports.)

But it doesn't explain why so many continue to maintain that the vaccines reduce transmission of the virus as well as offer protection to individuals—despite an abundance of evidence (both empirical and anecdotal) to the contrary.

One explanation may be found in an observation from economist Ludwig von Mises.

Mises famously observed that much of the strife in the modern world is a struggle over who designs the world, authorities or individuals. As Mises put it, we can either have "the democratic process of the market, in which every individual has his share, [or] the exclusive rule of a dictatorial body."

If getting vaccinated is simply a matter of individual health, there is little reason for "the planners" (as Mises called them) to exercise control over the public. It would be akin to requiring individuals to have cancerous tumors removed in the name of "public health."

But if not getting vaccinated is a threat to public health, or "society," then central planners have their reason (if not a valid justification) to exercise control over society.

In other words, evidence that shows COVID vaccination is primarily about individual health runs counter to the raison d'etre of the planners, which is to exercise their plan over society.

"What those calling themselves planners advocate is not the substitution of planned action for letting things go. It is the substitution of the planner's own plan for the plans of his fellow-men," Mises argued in Planned Chaos. "The planner is a potential dictator who wants to deprive all other people of the power to plan and act according to their own plans. He aims at one thing only: the exclusive absolute pre-eminence of his own plan."

For people trying to understand why for the first time in modern history public health officials are trying to combat a respiratory virus by coercing healthy individuals to take their desired actions—and in many cases lose their job and basic freedoms if they do not—Ludwig von Mises is required reading.

Periodical and Internet Sources Bibliography

The following articles have been selected to supplement the diverse views presented in this chapter.

Susan Brink, "Can't Help Falling in Love With a Vaccine: How Polio Campaign Beat Vaccine Hesitancy," NPR, May 3, 2021. https://news.virginia.edu/content/pediatrician-explains-how-covid-19-vaccines-kids-were-tested-safety.

Kathiann Kowalski, "Vaccines Help Everyone—Even the Unvaccinated," Science News for Students, April 4, 2019. https://www.sciencenewsforstudents.org/article/vaccines-help-everyone-even-unvaccinated.

Christopher Labos, M.D., MSc, "Natural Immunity to Covid Has Its Limits," McGill University, February 25, 2022. https://www.mcgill.ca/oss/article/covid-19/natural-immunity-covid-has-its-limits.

Nicoletta Lanese, "Why is the Flu Shot Less Effective Than Other Vaccines?" LIVESCIENCE, November 8, 2021. https://www.livescience.com/why-does-the-flu-shot-have-low-effectiveness.

John Ley, "Natural Immunity Gets Another Boost from Two New US Studies," Clark County Today, January 31, 2022. https://www.clarkcountytoday.com/news/natural-immunity-gets-another-boost-from-two-new-u-s-studies/.

Debbie Ann Shirley, "A Pediatrician Explains How Covid-19 Vaccines for Kids Were Tested for Safety," University of Virginia, November 1, 2021. https://news.virginia.edu/content/pediatrician-explains-how-covid-19-vaccines-kids-were-tested-safety.

Jocelyn Solis-Moreira, "What Causes Covid-19 Vaccine Side Effects?" LIVESCIENCE, April 1, 2021. https://www.livescience.com/what-causes-covid-19-vaccine-side-effects.html.

Melissa Suran, PhD, MSJ, "Why Parents Still Hesitate to Vaccinate Their Children Against Covid-19," JAMA Network, December 15, 2021. https://jamanetwork.com/journals/jama/fullarticle/2787289.

Opposing Viewpoints® Series

Chapter 2

Has the Media Affected the Acceptance of Vaccines?

Chapter Preface

Without a doubt, media affects the culture it inhabits. One could question whether the influence of media is good, bad, or neutral. Proponents and opponents could argue their point convincingly, while modern social media goes on and on pushing so-called "facts" that sometimes strain the boundaries of credibility. Viewing media through the lens of medicine and vaccines is challenging. Does social media push unverified falsehoods? Do people depend upon information from social media rather than seeking out medical truth from doctors and health professionals? Is social media contributing to outlandish conspiracy theories? Can social media be a vehicle of good when it comes to public health issues?

The viewpoints in this chapter explore the function of social media in the climate that has surrounded the COVID-19 timeframe with respect to vaccination. Some viewpoints in this chapter blame social media for increasing false information, while others show how doctors who are savvy with this modern communication modality can use it to counter false information. One viewpoint points out something that may be surprising—over half of the anti-vaccination sentiment is being pushed by a small number of people. Other viewpoints expose how entrenched conspiracy theories have become and how followers are attempting to go undercover to get around the social media companies trying to ban misinformation.

Not surprisingly, media affects the thinking and actions of some individuals. The viewpoint articles in this chapter debate and inform.

Viewpoint 1

> *"Social media platforms are usually free and accessible, and information is not vetted as with a news source."*

Social Media Facilitates the Spread of Misinformation

Katherine J. Igoe

In the following viewpoint Katherine J. Igoe analyzes the topic of social media and the spread of false information. Igoe asserts that there are really two types of false information that flourish on social media. Most people in the United States comply with vaccination protocols but don't advertise this on social media, thereby making the anti-vaccination adherents appear more numerous than they really are. Finally, Igoe outlines suggestions from experts on how anti-vaccination sentiment can be changed. Katherine J. Igoe is a freelance writer and editor.

As you read, consider the following questions:

1. What are the two types of false information that flourish on social media according to Igoe?
2. According to the viewpoint is there only one way to counter the spread of false information?

"Establishing the Truth: Vaccines, Social Media, and the Spread of Misinformation," by Katherine J. Igoe, Harvard T.H. Chan School of Public Health, July 10, 2019. Reprinted by permission.

3. Which community groups can effectively counter vaccine misinformation?

In June 2019, celebrity Jessica Biel lobbied against a pro-vaccine bill. She received intense backlash almost immediately, and the resulting scrutiny made international headlines. The exchange took place primarily on social media, where those against and those in favor of vaccines clashed—far from the first time such issues were aired loudly and publicly.

Vish Viswanath, Lee Kum Kee Professor of Health Communication and director of the Applied Risk Communication for the 21st Century program at the Harvard T.H. Chan School of Public Health, works to address this and other issues with social media and other platforms in the realm of public health. Such work focuses on the ways in which unverified information enters these popular platforms, and the impact of such information on public health. In order for public health professionals to understand how to combat these effects, they must first know the dangers of social media in relation to risk, and the effects these platforms have on large populations.

The Relationship Between Social Media and Public Health

Social media platforms are usually free and accessible, and information is not vetted as with a news source. "We always had writers and journalists as critical gatekeepers who were able to filter some of this information. But now, because of social media, we do not have this very critical intermediary," says Viswanath. Thus, social media has been proven to facilitate the spread of false information and risk.

There are two basic types of false information that flourish:

- Misinformation, or inadvertently drawing conclusions based on wrong or incomplete facts

- Disinformation, the deliberate spread of falsehoods to promote an agenda

The two are addressed differently—misinformation can be corrected with factual information but disinformation requires a different, more complex strategy.

Beyond public figures who use their fame to speak about subjects in which they are not experts, there are also social media influencers who spread and amplify inflammatory

Social Media's Impact on Vaccine Hesitancy

How do visuals on social media influence people's likelihood to get vaccinated?

Visuals on social media like memes, videos, photos, posters and emojis are processed faster, accepted without being questioned, and remembered for a longer period than text posts. Especially since the visual often includes a personalized dramatization of vaccine injuries—like an individual having a life-threatening seizure after receiving a vaccine.

Since social media has rapidly grown as a source of news, more and more people are obtaining health information from social media. As a result, visual messaging on social media has significant associations with people's intentions to get vaccinated—not only against COVID-19, but also for other immunizations. Specifically, our latest study has shown that individuals' engagement with anti-vaccine messages on social media has a negative impact on their intentions to get vaccinated, while their engagement with pro-vaccine messages has no significant association.

information through the social media megaphone. Social media can be a breeding ground for hate and intolerance around hot-button issues. Furthermore, activists can exploit fragile emotions of those impacted by the issue and provide misleading causal explanations.

"A large number of them are doing this anonymously: anonymity makes them uninhibited in expressing their opinions," explains Viswanath. The problem is compounded by "influence

How can social media users tell the difference between high quality vaccination information on social media and propaganda or misinformation?

Discerning accurate information from misinformation is a challenge that individuals may not be able to completely resolve. Social media puts us in a bubble called, "Echo chambers" where we are surrounded by like-minded individuals who reinforce our own existing views rather than being challenged by different views. Studies have shown that debiasing individuals especially from anti-vaccine beliefs is an extremely challenging task because health beliefs are deeply ingrained in our cultural backgrounds, political/religious beliefs and lifestyle choices. Thus, it is recommended to prevent populations that are especially vulnerable and susceptible to health misinformation from being exposed to it in the first place. It is essential to suppress the propagation of vaccine misinformation via social media. These solutions can be embedded in tools like fact-checkers installed in our web browsers that warn readers if the information to be presented is likely to be false.

"Ask the Expert: Social Media's Impact on Vaccine Hesitancy," MSU Today, June 15, 2021.

bots," anonymous, automated agents unattached to a real individual and sharing disinformation.

Treating the Source of Vaccine Misinformation

Vaccines are already a divisive topic, in part because the subject can be a very personal one. The blame, shame, and fear that can be inherent in parenthood, as well as the desire to protect one's child, are important aspects of understanding vaccine resistance.

The now-popular myth that vaccines cause autism comes from a simple mistake that's easy to make, according to Viswanath. "Most of us confuse correlation with causation. In general, a health care professional discovers symptoms of autism at about the same age period as when a child's undergoing immunization. Parents are genuinely struggling to make sense of what is happening to their kids, and they latch onto the explanation that's available to them. As a society, it's incumbent on us to be empathetic to parents who are going through this struggle."

Vaccine-resistant individuals have come to be known as "anti-vaxxers," but Viswanath believes this only creates more division. "Labeling only alienates people. We should be very careful how we categorize," he warns. In a similar way, providing purely scientific reasons for vaccinations without delving into the emotions and stories behind the reasoning is ineffective at driving change.

The Public Health Challenge of Communicating Vaccine Truth

Ironically, the vast majority of the U.S. public complies with vaccinations, but they don't speak up—leaving influencers to fill in the blank space with false information. "There has been some complacency. If you haven't seen polio in your life, you are not affected by it. Even if people who are against vaccinations are a very small group, they speak with a very amplified voice," Viswanath says.

Social media platforms themselves struggle with misinformation and disinformation—stuck between trying to find and address the problem, and existing within a democratic system that tolerates different beliefs. "The people who are spreading the information are always a few steps ahead—we are always in reactive mode," says Viswanath.

In May, Instagram announced that it would filter anti-vaccination misinformation (though they didn't specify when they would begin doing so). However, algorithms are not yet effective at allowing legitimate discussion while also blocking misinformation and disinformation effectively. Algorithms that are too wide-ranging might stifle legitimate questions and discussions. At this stage, they can only catch the most obvious instances of misinformation and disinformation.

An Effective Social Media Communications Strategy for Public Health Professionals

There's no magic bullet: no fail-safe, constantly successful tool that will always work against the spread of false information. "We need a multisectoral, multilevel strategy," explains Viswanath. "We want these platforms to take this seriously and put their resources and investments to minimize the problem as much as possible.

"We also have to equip our health care providers with resources to address these issues when they come up. More critical is to educate the parents right at the beginning even before these issues come up." Research has shown that when providers make recommendations on whether parents should vaccinate their children as a routine procedure, it helps parents feel comfortable trusting the professional. When doctors and professionals open it up for discussion, then parents can become hesitant or confused.

Understanding how vaccine resistance is reported and written about is another element of the strategy—giving voice to misinformation, even if the goal is to disprove it, can lead to more confusion. The better tactic is to starve it of oxygen, figuratively speaking, by not repeating the falsehood or giving validation to the person espousing it.

Doubling up on evidence-based, scientific communication strategies, and then tailoring the message to be most effective in each community, can be one of the most effective counterpoints to misinformation and disinformation.

"We have to work with community groups and organizations—schools, parent-teacher organizations, religious institutions—in making sure community norms include vaccinations and also counter the disinformation that is out there," Viswanath explains. "We don't want to wait for a crisis. And if one comes up, we want to have these relationships already in place to help."

Highlighting the manifold vaccine successes over time can remind the public of their impact—in other words, social media can also be a useful tool to provide real, factual information. For entities and corporations responsible for conveying this, the challenge is to present the truth neutrally, positively, and without blame. In other words, "We have to tone down the rhetoric, yet be proactive in promoting immunization," says Viswanath.

Viewpoint 2

> *"We have ... encouraged athletes to speak their mind on things. And, unfortunately, sometimes ... they're going to talk very wisely about issues that affect them, and, sometimes, they're going to quote Joe Rogan talking points."*

Celebrity Opinion on Vaccines Is Controversial

John Yang and Courtney Norris

In the following viewpoint, an interview with New York Magazine's Will Leitch, John Yang explores the role professional athletes have played in vaccine acceptancy. Though many professional athletes refused to receive the COVID vaccine, quarterback Aaron Rodgers was particularly criticized for his stance on the vaccine. John Yang is a correspondent for the PBS NewsHour. He reports on major national issues from Washington, DC, and across the country. Courtney Norris is a deputy senior producer of national affairs for the PBS NewsHour.

As you read, consider the following questions:

1. Why were Aaron Rodgers's remarks to reporters misleading?
2. Do the NBA and NFL have vaccination problems?

"What Aaron Rodgers' Controversy Tells Us About Vaccine Skepticism in Professional Sports," by John Yang and Courtney Norris, PBS NewsHour, November 12, 2021. Reproduced by permission of NewsHour Productions LLC.

3. What is a disadvantage of deep player engagement, as evidenced by Aaron Rodgers and Kyrie Irving, according to the viewpoint?

Will Leitch, a contributing editor for New York Magazine, and John Yang discuss the controversy over Green Bay Packers quarterback Aaron Rodgers' vaccination status. Rodgers had previously implied he was inoculated against COVID-19, but later admitted to being unvaccinated after contracting the virus.

John Yang: Speaking with reporters in August, Green Bay Packers quarterback Aaron Rodgers implied he was inoculated against COVID-19.

Question: Are you vaccinated? And what's your stance on vaccinations?

Aaron Rodgers, Green Bay Packers: Yes, I have been immunized. There's guys on the team that haven't been vaccinated. I think it's a personal decision. I'm not going to judge those guys.

John Yang: But after testing positive, the reigning league MVP was in required isolation for last Sunday's game against the Kansas City Chiefs.

On Pat McAfee's satellite radio show last week, Rodgers acknowledged he is not vaccinated.

Aaron Rodgers: I believe strongly in bodily autonomy and the ability to make choices for your body.

John Yang: Rodgers said he has concerns about all three federally approved vaccines, and was denied league approval for an alternative treatment, which he said he underwent in consultation with Joe Rogan, the talk show host and prominent vaccine skeptic.

This week, Rodgers was back on McAfee's show with a different play.

Aaron Rodgers: I made some comments that people may have felt were misleading. And to anybody who felt misled by those comments, I take full responsibility.

John Yang: Rodgers is one of a handful of high-profile professional athletes who have either declined to get vaccinated or be fully forthcoming about their status, in spite of league rules and local vaccine mandates.

Brooklyn Nets point guard Kyrie Irving has yet to play a game this season because New York City requires anyone entering an indoor arena to show proof of vaccination, and the team won't use him only in games out of the city.

Steve Nash, Brooklyn Nets Head Coach: I support the decision. And if things change, we'd love to have Kyrie back.

John Yang: Rodgers is paying a price. A Green Bay-based health care provider, Prevea Health, ended its nine-year partnership him, saying it "remains deeply committed to protecting its patients, staff, providers, and communities amidst the COVID-19 pandemic. This includes encouraging and helping all eligible populations to become vaccinated against COVID-19."

And this week, the NFL fined Rodgers $14, 650 for breaking league rules by not wearing a mask when talking with reporters and attending an event with other players outside team facilities. The Packers were fined $300,000 for not policing his behavior.

Rodgers could be cleared to play in this Sunday's game against the Seattle Seahawks.

Will Leitch is a contributing editor for "New York Magazine" and has been writing about the issue.

Will, thanks for joining us.

So many people are talking about the Rodgers case, not just football fans, but sort of casual football fans. Why do you think Aaron Rodgers' case is resonating so much?

Will Leitch, "New York Magazine": Well, Aaron Rodgers, in a lot of ways, was a quarterback that I think a lot of people thought they knew.

And I think—remember, he was—had offered to take off a year of in play in the NFL to host "Jeopardy," not something you generally would assume someone who would be a vaccine skeptic. He was like—he's very outgoing. He's very open on social media. He's actually been actually quite seeming progressive on some topics.

He was very eloquent during the racial protests last summer of, like, really talking about kind of supporting social justice. And for a lot of people, I think there was a notion that Rodgers was the smart quarterback and was the one that was somewhat—was very ahead of the game and very kind of the quarterback that was maybe different from what people fairly or unfairly will consider like a dumb jock stereotype.

And I think he's on the State Farm ads. He's funny in those ads. He was a good "Jeopardy" host.

John Yang: You know, we mentioned the fine, $14,000. We should also note that he is in the second year of a four-year $134 million contract.

The same week, the NFL fined a Cowboys player, CeeDee Lamb, for wearing an untucked uniform. That fine was $20,000. What do you make of that?

Will Leitch: Well, on one hand, I think what—the Packers were also, of course, fined for not having some of the protocols in place.

I think it's not actually—you don't have to be vaccinated to play in the NFL. I think that's been a little lost a little bit. And I also think the idea that there are more—I think people think there are more unvaccinated players in the NFL than they are.

Rodgers didn't break any rules by not being vaccinated. But by not wearing the mask, it was a minor thing in generally the way the Packers kind of run the program. But I think what was really the issue, and I think why they didn't fine him too much is, basically, what he did was he deceived people, which—and, frankly, deceive people in a press conference, which I will say, if the NFL started fining people for that, there would be a lot of fines, I would say.

I think that the protocols he generally—the team is the one that is seen to have not adhered by the protocols. Remember, the team surely knew that he was not vaccinated. The NFL surely knew that he was not vaccinated.

John Yang: And talking about the other—the instance with Kyrie Irving, the NBA commissioner, Adam Silver, has said he would prefer to have a vaccine mandate, but the players union objected.

What does that say about the—sort of the balance of power in professional sports these days?

Will Leitch: I think that player unions are wary of any sort of management having any extra power over labor than they already do.

And so I certainly understand that in a macro sense. A lot of players will argue—and, frankly, leagues will argue this as well—in a lot of ways, the NFL and the NBA don't have vaccination problems. The NBA has 96 percent of its players vaccinated. The NFL has 95 percent of its players vaccinated.

I have to tell you, you or I should feel so fortunate to walk around, to be around 95 or 96 percent of people vaccinated. It's these high-profile cases like Rodgers, like Irving that make people think that there is some sort of larger issue.

They're—I think the leaks would argue, and I think fairly, that they have not actually had mandates, but have still had buy-in to a degree that's much higher than the general population. And I think, when people like Rodgers—people think that, like, oh, here's this NFL player or Irving, this NBA player, what's—why is there a vaccine resistance in sports?

There really kind of isn't. It's just when—these high-profile things, it makes it look like there is.

John Yang: And in his high-profile response, Aaron Rodgers hit sort of hit all the hot buttons. He talked about cancel culture. He talked about woke mobs. He talked about a media witch-hunt.

And you also talked about how he had been on sort of racial justice and Black Lives Matter, and how Kyrie Irving had been on Black Lives Matter. Is this—in some sense, could this be seen as a logical extension of players speaking out on social issues?

Will Leitch: Certainly, I do think that this is the age of player empowerment in a lot of ways. And there are a lot of positives to that.

I think that we have really spent a lot of the last year-and-a-half saying, listen to athletes. They have stories to tell. They're from communities that have been overlooked for a long time. This is certainly a downside to that, in that there is influence that these athletes have.

To be fair, they have always had this sort of influence. I would love—like, Charles Barkley famously, years ago said, "I'm not a role model."

But we have kind of encouraged athletes to speak their mind on things. And, unfortunately, sometimes, they're going to be eloquent, and, sometimes, they're going to talk very wisely about issues that affect them, and, sometimes, they're going to quote Joe Rogan talking points.

So, I think that there is a downside to that. I think the thing with Rodgers, and I think the reason his has resonated so much, it really feels like a surprise. It really feels like we have learned something about an athlete that we thought we knew, and it's very different than the perception we had of that athlete.

John Yang: Will Leitch of "New York Magazine," thank you very much.

Will Leitch: My pleasure. Thanks for having me.

Viewpoint 3

> *"...12 people are responsible for the bulk of the misleading claims and outright lies about COVID-19 vaccines that proliferate on Facebook, Instagram and Twitter."*

Over Half of Vaccine Misinformation on Social Media Is Produced by Only 12 People

Shannon Bond

In the following viewpoint Shannon Bond presents a startling accusation—that only 12 people are responsible for producing over half of the vaccine misinformation spreading over social media platforms. Bond analyzes this assertion and explains some of the tactics used by these twelve purveyors of falsities. Bond also outlines some of the ways that social media sites are attempting to lessen the impact from misinformation. Shannon Bond is a business correspondent at NPR and most often writes about technology and Silicon Valley.

As you read, consider the following questions:

1. According to the viewpoint, is modern vaccine misinformation new?
2. Which well known American is one of the Disinformation Dozen?

©2021 National Public Radio, Inc. NPR news report titled "Just 12 People Are Behind Most Vaccine Hoaxes on Social Media, Research Shows" by Shannon Bond was originally published on npr.org on May 14, 2021, and is used with the permission of NPR. Any unauthorized duplication is strictly prohibited.

3. What is one way the Disinformation Dozen uses to get around social media rules?

Researchers have found just 12 people are responsible for the bulk of the misleading claims and outright lies about COVID-19 vaccines that proliferate on Facebook, Instagram and Twitter.

"The 'Disinformation Dozen' produce 65% of the shares of anti-vaccine misinformation on social media platforms," said Imran Ahmed, chief executive officer of the Center for Countering Digital Hate, which identified the accounts.

Now the vaccine rollout is reaching a critical stage in which most adults who want the vaccine have gotten it, but many others are holding out, these 12 influential social media users stand to have an outsize impact on the outcome.

After this story published on Thursday, Facebook said it had taken down more of the accounts run by these 12 individuals.

These figures are well-known to both researchers and the social networks. They include anti-vaccine activists, alternative health entrepreneurs and physicians. Some of them run multiple accounts across the different platforms. They often promote "natural health." Some even sell supplements and books.

Many of the messages about the COVID-19 vaccines being widely spread online mirror what's been said in the past about other vaccines by peddlers of health misinformation.

"It's almost like conspiracy theory Mad Libs. They just inserted the new claims," said John Gregory, deputy health editor at NewsGuard, which rates the credibility of news sites and has done its own tracking of COVID-19 and vaccine misinformation "superspreaders."

The claims from the "Disinformation Dozen" range from "denying that COVID exists, claiming that false cures are in fact the way to solve COVID and not vaccination, decrying vaccines and decrying doctors as being in some way venal or motivated by other factors when they recommend vaccines," Ahmed said.

Many of the 12, he said, have been spreading scientifically disproven medical claims and conspiracies for years.

Which provokes the question: Why have social media platforms only recently begun cracking down on their falsehoods?

Both members of Congress and state attorneys general have urged Facebook and Twitter to ban the "Disinformation Dozen."

"Getting Americans vaccinated is critical to putting this pandemic behind us. Vaccine disinformation spread online has deadly consequences, which is why I have called on social media platforms to take action against the accounts propagating the majority of these lies," Sen. Amy Klobuchar, D-Minn., told NPR.

Social Networks Crack Down on COVID-19 Vaccine Claims

The companies have stopped short of taking all 12 figures offline entirely, but they have stepped up their fight: They've labeled misleading posts. They've removed falsehoods. In some cases, they've banned people who repeatedly share debunked claims.

After NPR's reporting, Facebook said it had taken additional action against some of the figures identified by the Center for Countering Digital Hate, several of which operate multiple accounts on the social network's apps. The company said on Thursday it had found new posts violating its rules.

Facebook has now removed 16 accounts from Facebook or Instagram and placed restrictions on 22 others, such as preventing them from being recommended to other users, reducing the reach of their posts and blocking them from promoting themselves through paid ads.

"We reacted early and aggressively to the COVID-19 pandemic by working with health experts to update our misinformation policy to target harmful claims about COVID-19 and vaccines, including taking action against some of the accounts in the CCDH report," spokesperson Kevin McAlister said in a statement. "In total, we've removed more than 16 million pieces of content which violate our policies and we continue to work with health experts to regularly update these policies as new facts and trends emerge."

However, Facebook also disputed the methodology of the center's report, saying it was not clear what criteria the group used to choose the set of social media posts at which it looked.

Twitter said it permanently suspended two of the "Disinformation Dozen" accounts for repeatedly breaking its rules, required other accounts to delete some tweets and applied labels that link to credible information about vaccines and don't allow the tweets to be shared or replied to. Overall, it's removed more than 22,400 tweets for violating its COVID-19 policies.

However, spokesperson Elizabeth Busby said Twitter distinguishes between "harmful vaccine misinformation that contradicts credible public health information, which is prohibited under our policy, and negative vaccine sentiment that is a matter of opinion."

And so the "Disinformation Dozen" are still easy to find on social media.

"Tried and True" Tactics

Sometimes they skirt the platforms' rules by using codes.

"Instead of saying 'vaccine,' they may, in a video, hold up the V sign with their fingers and say, 'If you're around someone who has been'—hold up V sign—'you know, X might happen to you,' " Ahmed said.

Or they take something true and distort it, such as falsely linking a famous person's death to the fact that the celebrity got a vaccine days or weeks earlier.

NewsGuard's Gregory said a "tried and true" tactic of vaccine opponents is "grossly misrepresenting some sort of research, some sort of data to promote whatever narrative they've chosen."

Facebook said it now limits the reach of posts that could discourage people from getting vaccinated, even if the messages don't explicitly break its rules.

But the cat-and-mouse game continues.

Anti-Vaccine Activists Claim Censorship

As the social networks have cracked down, some previously prolific spreaders of vaccine misinformation have toned down their posts and have told their followers they are being censored.

Take anti-vaccine activist Robert F. Kennedy Jr., one of the "Disinformation Dozen" identified by the center, who has promoted the long discredited idea that vaccines are linked to autism. During the pandemic, he has shared baseless conspiracy theories linking 5G cellular networks to the coronavirus, and suggested, without evidence, that the death of baseball great Hank Aaron was "part of a wave of suspicious deaths" tied to vaccines.

None of that is true.

Kennedy was kicked off Instagram, which Facebook owns, in February over repeatedly sharing debunked claims.

Yet Facebook did not remove him from its namesake platform. He told NPR the company has flagged some of his posts, however, so he has become more cautious.

"I have to post, like, unicorns and kitty cat pictures on there," he said. "I don't want to give them an excuse."

He also uses it to promote his website and newsletter, where he makes claims he cannot on the social network.

Kennedy said he's never posted misinformation and accused Facebook of censorship. He said the crackdown has cost "hundreds of thousands of dollars" in donations to his organization.

A Battle of Persuasion

Even as the social media companies have gotten tougher recently on misinformation, researchers worry the persistence of vaccine-related hoaxes will further erode confidence among people who hesitate to get the shot.

That's especially concerning as vaccines roll out for children 12 and up.

In a survey of U.S parents, Indiana University sociologist Jessica Calarco found more than a quarter don't plan to vaccinate their kids.

"So many of these moms are turning to Facebook, are turning to Twitter, are turning to other social media platforms" for news and information, she said. "And they're saying, 'Every time I open my phone, I see something different.'"

Even some parents whose kids have had routine childhood vaccines told Calarco they're unsure about COVID-19 jabs.

Facebook this week released survey data showing vaccine acceptance among adults in the U.S. has increased by 10% since January. However, its survey also shows that the top reasons people said they don't want to get vaccinated are worries about side effects and lack of trust in the vaccines or the government—exactly the kind of fears anti-vaccination accounts promote.

The social networks said amplifying credible information from authoritative sources, such as the Centers for Disease Control and Prevention, is just as important as reducing the spread of harmful posts. Both Facebook and Twitter link to public health information in their apps and in the labels they put on misleading posts.

But they now face an uphill battle of persuading the skeptics.

Calarco said many of the parents she spoke with weigh the posts they see on social media "equally against the kinds of expert medical recommendations, expert medical information coming out of things like the CDC."

Viewpoint 4

> *"Q-Anon weaves a myriad of conspiracies, from anti-vaccine and anti-5G conspiracies to antisemitic and antimigrant tropes."*

Anti-Vaccine Conspiracy Theories Are Easy to Promote via QAnon

Ian M. Haimovitz

In the following viewpoint Ian M. Haimovitz spotlights how the conspiracy theory QAnon got started, how it can negatively impact factual health information, and potentially how its hold on people may be stopped. Haimovitz outlines the outlandish claims of QAnon and how an innocent user of social media may be sucked into a vortex of conspiratorial lies, which in some instances has become violent. Additionally, Haimovitz reports on the ways that social media companies are trying to combat QAnon. Ian M. Haimovitz is a former visiting fellow with the Strategic Technologies Program at the Center for Strategic and International Studies in Washington, DC.

As you read, consider the following questions:

1. According to Haimovitz, what is the root of QAnon?
2. What conspiracies does QAnon promote?

"No One is Immune: The Spread of Q-Anon Through Social Media and the Pandemic," by Ian M. Haimowitz, Center for Strategic and International Studies, December 17, 2020. Reprinted by permission.

3. How have social media companies tried to work against QAnon?

At some point, you were exposed—and probably also fascinated—by a conspiracy theory. Conspiracy theories are not a new phenomenon. From Ancient Aliens, to pondering if there was another shooter on the grassy knoll, our brains intuitively look for patterns to process information, despite that "sometimes a cigar is just a cigar" as Sigmund Freud noted. However, with most of our attention directed online due to the pandemic, and the rising prevalence of the anti-vaccination and anti-mask movements, we must reexamine how outlandish theories are spreading across the social media ecosystem. Q-Anon, a far-right conspiracy theory, is an example of how a conspiracy theory can change and spread through the power of the internet.

Q-Anon is rooted in the idea that an elite group of child-trafficking pedophiles has been ruling the world, from Hollywood elites to senior Democratic political figures. The conspiracy traces back to October 28, 2017, when a user from the messaging board 4chan—an anonymous online forum considered the "ninth circle of hell" due to its constant appeal for outrage—revealed the first "Q Drop." Q, the predominant spokesperson of these conspiracies, claims to have a high-level security clearance that has allowed him/her to access this information. Never mind that Q clearances belong to the Department of Energy, equivalent to a Top-Secret clearance that provides access to restricted data on nuclear weapons and facilities, not pedophiles (the exact relations of Q to the Department of Energy is not known at this time). The Q drops, riddled with cryptic language and peppered with slogans and pledges, captures the story of Donald Trump's role in saving the world from pedophiles.

Q successfully brought attention to his fight against the "deep state." For example, the #ReleaseTheMemo campaign, a push for the release of Rep. David Nunes's intelligence memorandum detailing missing FBI text messages to "imaginary secret societies plotting internal coups against the president" saw a 233,000% increase in tweets with the related hashtag in less than 48 hours. While some report that this was achieved thanks to the amplification of Russian bots, since 2018 the Q-Anon conspiracy has spread, pouring into the physical world. Q-Anon conspiracies have been the cause of several violent attacks, including breaking into the residence of the Canadian prime minister, an armed standoff near the Hoover dam, and several kidnapping plots, with two successful kidnappings.

To facilitate its spread, Q-Anon weaves a myriad of conspiracies, from anti-vaccine and anti-5G conspiracies to antisemitic and antimigrant tropes. Social media algorithms, designed to maximize user engagement, make this easier. If you are, for example, into yoga, your Facebook ads and recommendations will be tailored around that interest; maybe suggesting some essential oil groups. It is in these groups that conspiracy theorists thrive, with posts about a variety of issues populating the feed. It's not hard to imagine articles on anxieties related to vaccinations getting some traction, appealing to new members. What was initially a harmless search into non-traditional healing practices, with the help of algorithms and misinformation, has blurred reality, and convinced users that essential oils can replace vaccines. Intentionally or not, social media is creating a pipeline to conspiracy theories.

Yoga-enthusiast turned anti-vaxxer may sound extreme, but this method has been co-opted by Q-Anon to conscript new supporters, while also leading to vaccination rates as low as "Chad or South Sudan" in certain communities. According to researchers like Mia Bloom, a professor at Georgia State University and a leading expert in radicalization, there has been a 174% increase in Q-Anon posts throughout the Covid-19 pandemic. Such messaging is attempting to do the same as the yoga example, exploiting anxieties attributed to governmental overreach (mask mandates), economic disruption (lockdowns), and other areas (anti-vax and government microchips).

Facebook has de-platformed groups associated with Q-Anon, gradually banning all pages, groups, and Instagram accounts.

However, efforts have been slow, with only 790 groups removed earlier in 2020, showing the new difficulties in limiting this group. Twitter is said to have changed its algorithm to stop recommending Q-Anon related accounts and trends, however there are still over 93,000 active accounts referencing Q-Anon. Other technology platforms are attempting to circumnavigate how to limit Q-anon without completely banning it.

However, when one post is taken down, there still may be ten unnoticed, as individuals within Q are told to "deploy camouflage" to avoid any "censorship." So instead of using #QAnon on their social media posts, they now use #SavetheChildren. Such efforts are what researcher Marc-André Argentino calls "pastel Q," an attempt to make Q theories more palatable to the general population, to begin their algorithmic descent into conspiracy theories.

While once a fringe movement, Q-Anon's growth is exponential, with 22,232,285 tweets with #QAnon or related hashtags in 2019. Comparatively, other popular hashtags in 2019 have less than half the tweets, with #MeToo at 5,231,928 tweets and #climatechange at 7,510,311. Likewise, Q has spread throughout the world. The United States, U.K., Canada, Australia, and Germany account for the top five countries producing Q-Anon tweets, and of 150 Telegram groups (one of the leading methods of Q communications), 84 were in German. The international spread of Q is using the interconnectivity of the internet to grow new appendages. However, while the main focus on Q is to stop the cabal of elites battling Trump, the conspiracy theory has been localized to different countries, adding unique twists. In Japan, the conspiracies have included local issues, whether complaints that the Prime Minister's media ratings are inflated, to even suggesting that a Japanese movie, "Demon Slayer: Kimetsu no Yaiba," is warning the Japanese people of the pedophilia and cannibalism of the international elite. According to Graphika, a social media analytics firm, Q has diverged, with Brazil and Japan leading the localized efforts, and Western Europe mirroring the U.S. version, while still including their own respective governments.

Fighting Q-Anon's capture of minds requires a new approach One alternative is to implement "off-ramping" measures, originally a method to disengage and deradicalize individuals from violent extremism. Instead of attempting to prevent someone from entering the pipeline of conspiracy theories, the focus is to prevent such efforts from becoming violent. In this case, efforts can come from social media companies by providing access to new networks. Meaning while someone is interested in yoga, and has metaphorically drank the Kool-Aid, companies can recommend knitting instead. While knitting might not be the solution for everybody, it is necessary to remember Albert Camus's words: In order to understand the world, one has to turn away from it on occasion. Perhaps social media companies could encourage people to take a break from their algorithmic deluge of conspiracies. If not, there are risks of harmless scrolling on the internet turning into violent actions against innocent people.

Viewpoint 5

> *"More scholarly study and new strategies are needed from public health and other arms of government to counter these anti-vaccination cults."*

Anti-Vaxx Cults Must Be Minimized with the Help of Media

Healthy Debate

In the following viewpoint Healthy Debate argues that anti-vaxx enthusiasts have become a cult. The author maintains that many of these individuals may actually be displacing their disagreements with governments and governmental mandates with anti-vaxx sentiment. Either way, the author insists that anti-vaxx cults must be dealt with and minimized. Healthy Debate publishes journalism about health care in Canada by the people whose lives it touches the most, from physicians, patients and caregivers to health journalists, academics, and advocates.

As you read, consider the following questions:

1. According to the author how do media bolster anti-vaxxers?
2. How could the media aid public health experts in the fight against anti-vaxx setiment?
3. What is one characteristic of cults as stated in the viewpoint?

"Enough with the Harassment: How to Deal With Anti-Vax Cults," Healthy Debate, January 26, 2022. https://healthydebate.ca/2022/01/topic/how-to-deal-with-anti-vax-cults/. Licensed under CC BY-ND 4.0 International.

Anti-vax protesters arrived at my home recently. I am not unique in having experienced this; many medical officers of health and civil servants have throughout the pandemic. I started in my current role recently, so although I have explicitly taken a strong position of no-tolerance of harassment against my staff and actively dispelling misinformation circulating from our community, this escalation was disconcerting.

It was suggested that my condemnation of protests obstructing our facility were in part to blame for the actions brought to my home over the weekend. Indeed, one sign affixed to my house read: "You didn't like our protest at (the public health office) so … here we are!"

The protesters' tactics are evidently intended to harass and intimidate, and suggesting that protests were brought to my home because of my strong public position amounts to victim-blaming. I also recognize that softening my strong public position in response may put wind in their sails as the groups sense Pyrrhic victory.

Having trained and worked in public health, I have learned our 3 Cs framework for vaccine uptake: complacency, convenience and confidence. Sometimes a fourth C is added, culture, but given my observations perhaps cult is a more appropriate framing for the present issues.

Increasingly, I am noting that the anti-vaxxers we are dealing with visibly in the public and bolstered by continuous media attention, those protesting at our hospitals and at my own home, demonstrate a cult-like phenomenon and are conflating broad antagonism with the system and government with anti-vaccination (and anti-lockdown, anti-mask) rhetoric.

As one individual wrote in social media comments related to the protesters at my house: "They don't even care about the vaccines … This is just a social club for local assholes." Some individuals may not deeply believe in what they spew or may be hypocritical in their personal decisions. These cults are also conflating broad disgruntlement with the pandemic and its restrictions on liberty with anti-vaccination. The media attention they garner and the messages they spread impact vaccine confidence for the rest of the population and may cause lasting damage to vaccine programs.

More scholarly study and new strategies are needed from public health and other arms of government to counter these anti-vaccination cults.

Firstly, we need to actively work with media for responsible reporting and avoid giving disproportionate voice to this vocal minority. This means supporting responsible journalism. Public health physicians or other vaccine experts must be as available and responsive to media inquiries as possible. It may mean bolstering pre-pandemic communications capacity given the heightening demands for information placed on our public health organizations.

Secondly, we need to counter vaccine misinformation rhetoric with strong public health messaging because if their loud rhetoric is not countered, it will impact confidence in the broader public. As Peter Hotez, dean of the National School of Tropical Medicine at Baylor College of Medicine and co-director of the Texas Children's Hospital Center for Vaccine Development, has written: "The bad guys are winning, in part because health agencies either underestimate or deny the reach of anti-science forces and are ill-equipped to counter it." The common wisdom to "not vocally counter it" because it "adds fuel to the fire" represents a misunderstanding of the scope of the current problem. It also represents a misunderstanding of the principles of forest fire management. Sometimes directly and strongly countering with "a controlled burn" is healthier for the forest as a whole. This is, however, difficult to implement when you are targeted personally.

Thirdly, we need to consider that while much traditional vaccine hesitancy induced by internet misinformation exists, some anti-vaxxer groups now conform to cult-like characteristics. We must therefore learn from sociology's study of the phenomenon. They form and multiply on social media. Cult characteristics include the seeking of loyalty to their leaders, opposing critical thinking and the same messaging rhetoric to indoctrinate their followers. We therefore need to learn from sociology on the practices for therapy and support for exiting cults that have been effective in other domains.

Fourthly, we need to ensure that public health workers, such as myself, are personally supported in their work and personally protected from these groups through strong and effective implementation of the amendments to the criminal code to counter health-care protests through Bill C-3. Provincial legislation prohibiting protests near health facilities, such as Quebec's Law 105, is also important.

Anti-vaxxers are becoming a liability to our pandemic exit strategy. They influence broader individuals who are only vaccine hesitant. We need to act urgently before more individuals are recruited, their support base grows and confidence in vaccines and public health more broadly erodes further.

Periodical and Internet Sources Bibliography

The following articles have been selected to supplement the diverse views presented in this chapter.

Shannon Bond, "Unwelcome on Facebook and Twitter, QAnon Followers Flock to Fringe Sites," NPR, January 31, 2021. https://www.npr.org/2021/01/31/962104747/unwelcome-on-facebook-twitter-qanon-followers-flock-to-fringe-sites.

Talha Burki, "Vaccine Misinformation and Social Media," *The Lancet*, October 1, 2019. https://www.thelancet.com/journals/landig/article/PIIS2589-7500(19)30136-0/fulltext.

Sarah Dawood, "From QAnon to Anti-Vaxx: Can You Cure a Conspiracy Theorist?" *New Statesman*, March 14, 2020. https://www.newstatesman.com/spotlight/cyber/2022/03/conspiracy-theories-online-psychology.

Elizabeth Dwoskin and Isaac Stanley-Becker, "Facebook Says it Will Crack Down on QAnon Conspiracy Theory But Stops Short of Full Ban," *Washington Post*, August 19, 2020. https://www.washingtonpost.com/technology/2020/08/19/facebook-crackdown-qanon/.

Sheera Frenkel and Tiffany Hsu, "How Local Media Spreads Misinformation From Vaccine Skeptics," *New York Times*, August 1, 2021. https://www.nytimes.com/2021/08/01/technology/local-media-misinformation-vaccine-skeptics.html.

Darcy Jimenez, "Covid-19 Vaccines: The Role of Social Media in Disinformation," Pharmaceutical Technology, June 4, 2021. https://www.pharmaceutical-technology.com/features/covid-19-vaccine-disinformation-social-media/.

Amy Mitchell and Jacob Liedke, "About Four-in-Ten Americans Say Social Media is an Important Way of Following Covid-19 Vaccine News," Pew Research Center, August 24, 2021. https://www.pewresearch.org/fact-tank/2021/08/24/about-four-in-ten-americans-say-social-media-is-an-important-way-of-following-covid-19-vaccine-news/.

Kevin Roose, "YouTube Cracks Down on QAnon Conspiracy Theory, Citing Offline Violence," *New York Times*, September 29, 2021.

https://www.nytimes.com/2020/10/15/technology/youtube-bans-qanon-violence.html.

Anjana Susarla, "Big Tech Has a Vaccine Misinformation Problem—Here's What a Social Media Expert Recommends," The Conversation, July 29, 2021. https://theconversation.com/big-tech-has-a-vaccine-misinformation-problem-heres-what-a-social-media-expert-recommends-164987.

Craig Timberg and Elizabeth Dwoskin, "With Trump Gone, QAnon Groups Focus Fury on Attacking Coronavirus Vaccines," *Washington Post*, March 11, 2021. https://www.washingtonpost.com/technology/2021/03/11/with-trump-gone-qanon-groups-focus-fury-attacking-covid-vaccines/.

Brandy Zadrozny, "Anti-Vaccination Groups Target Local Media After Social Media Crackdowns," NBC News, December 17, 2020. https://www.nbcnews.com/tech/tech-news/anti-vaccination-groups-target-local-media-after-social-media-crackdowns-n1251485.

OPPOSING VIEWPOINTS® SERIES

Chapter 3

Does Politics Alter the Perception of Vaccines in Society?

Chapter Preface

People vehemently disagreeing with each other. Families divided over political ideals. Local government officials quitting because of intense and sometimes violent squabbling over issues. School board officials receiving threats to themselves and family members. It appears that civility and the ability to have an opinion opposed to others are no longer tolerated among many in the U.S. And this lack of empathy and escalating political rhetoric spills over into people's feelings surrounding vaccines.

Why is it that an individual's political affiliation should color their beliefs when it comes to science, medicine, and vaccinations? After all, vaccines are developed to fight off viruses and the illness they cause. Disease affects everyone and doesn't discriminate between people of differing political affiliations. So, what is the correlation between political affiliation and vaccine understanding and beliefs?

This chapter's viewpoints cast a spotlight on these issues. Obviously, there are politically identifiable groups that appear to support science and vaccination, while others seem to mistrust scientific experts and government officials. Not surprisingly, there are some individuals that insist it is their right to not get vaccinated because of individual autonomy. Some people, whether sincerely or not, claim that their religion prohibits using vaccines. And then there are other, seeming outliers that defy categorization. The authors of the viewpoints that follow debate these topics.

Viewpoint 1

> *"Democrats are far more likely than Republicans to have received at least one COVID-19 vaccine dose, though majorities in both groups say they have done so."*

Political Affiliation Affects Americans' Views on Coronavirus Vaccines

Cary Funk and John Gramlich

In the following viewpoint Cary Funk and John Gramlich analyze the factors affecting American's views on the COVID-19 vaccine. As outlined in their report, the authors present several factors, including political affiliation, that appear to affect how individuals feel about the vaccine. Funk and Gramlich maintain that politics, religion, race, education and a level of confusion affect how Americans view the coronavirus vaccine. Cary Funk is a director of science research at the Pew Research Center. John Gramlich is a senior writer and editor at the Pew Research Center.

As you read, consider the following questions:

1. How does strict party affiliation affect a person's view of the vaccine as stated in the viewpoint?
2. How does education affect personal vaccine choice?
3. How does party affiliation affect personal views about the U.S. helping other nations obtain COVID vaccinations?

"10 Facts About Americans and Coronavirus Vaccines," by Cary Funk and John Gramlich, Pew Research Center, September 20, 2021.

The coronavirus pandemic has claimed more than 670,000 lives in the United States as of Sept. 20, and the spread of the highly transmissible delta variant has added new urgency to the federal government's efforts to vaccinate all Americans against the virus. As the drive to inoculate more people continues, here are 10 facts about Americans and COVID-19 vaccines, based on an August Pew Research Center survey of more than 10,000 U.S. adults.

1.

Around three-quarters of U.S. adults (73%) said in August that they had received at least one dose of a COVID-19 vaccine, with the vast majority in this group saying they were fully vaccinated. The survey findings align closely with administrative data from the Centers of Disease Control and Prevention, which, as of early September, showed that three-quarters of adults had received at least one vaccine dose. Surveys have generally aligned closely with the CDC's vaccination data.

2.

Democrats are far more likely than Republicans to have received at least one COVID-19 vaccine dose, though majorities in both groups say they have done so. Among Democrats and independents who lean to the Democratic Party, 86% said they were at least partially vaccinated as of August, compared with six-in-ten Republicans and GOP leaners. Factoring in ideology as well as party affiliation, nine-in-ten self-described liberal Democrats said they had received at least one dose, compared with 83% of conservative or moderate Democrats, 63% of moderate or liberal Republicans and 58% of conservative Republicans.

3.

In both parties, older people and those with higher levels of education are more likely to have received at least one dose. As of August, 86% of Americans ages 65 and older said they were at least partially vaccinated, compared with 73% of those ages

50 to 64, 69% of those 30 to 49 and 66% of those 18 to 29. Older Americans were among the first groups to become eligible for COVID-19 vaccines due to the increased risk of severe illness they face from the virus.

Americans with more formal schooling are also more likely to be vaccinated. Around nine-in-ten of those with a postgraduate degree or more (89%) said they had received at least one dose by August, compared with smaller shares of those with a bachelor's degree (81%), some college education (69%) or a high school diploma or less (66%).

These patterns appear in both partisan coalitions. Among Republicans, for example, 80% of those ages 65 and older said they had received at least one dose by August—far higher than the share of younger Republicans who had done so.

4.

Unlike earlier in the pandemic, Black and White adults are about equally likely to say they have been vaccinated. Around seven-in-ten Black and White Americans (70% and 72%, respectively) said they had received at least one vaccine dose as of August. Earlier in the outbreak, Black adults were less likely than White adults to say they planned to get a COVID-19 vaccine or had already done so.

Other major racial and ethnic groups also reported high vaccination rates in the August survey. Around three-quarters of Hispanic adults (76%) said they were at least partially vaccinated, as did 94% of Asian adults. It's important to note, however, that Asian adults were surveyed in English only and may not necessarily be representative of all Asian Americans.

5.

Vaccination patterns vary considerably among major U.S. religious groups. Around eight-in-ten Catholic adults (82%) said they were at least partially vaccinated as of August—a figure that included 86% of Hispanic Catholics and 79% of White Catholics. Among Protestants, 73% of White non-evangelicals and 70% of those who are Black said they had received at least dose, but the share was considerably lower among White evangelical Protestants (57%).

When it comes to religiously unaffiliated Americans, three-quarters said they were at least partially vaccinated as of August. But there were differences within this group too: Nine-in-ten atheists said they had received at least one dose, compared with somewhat smaller shares of agnostics (84%) and those who describe their religion as "nothing in particular" (69%).

6.

Vaccination status is strongly linked with confidence in the vaccine research and development process. Around nine-in-ten adults who were at least partially vaccinated as of August (91%) said they had a great deal or fair amount of confidence in the vaccine R&D process, compared with only 21% of those who were not vaccinated. Only 3% of unvaccinated adults said they had a great deal of confidence in the vaccine R&D process.

7.

Americans who are not inoculated against COVID-19 express a range of concerns about the vaccines. The August survey asked Americans whether various statements about COVID-19 vaccines describe them very well, somewhat well, not too well or not at all well. At least eight-in-ten unvaccinated adults said the following statements describe them very or somewhat well: "There's too much pressure on Americans to get a COVID-19 vaccine" (88%); "We don't really know yet if there are serious health risks from COVID-19 vaccines" (81%); and "Public health officials are not telling us everything they know about COVID-19 vaccines" (80%). Seven-in-ten unvaccinated adults also said the following statement describes them very or somewhat well: "It's hard to make sense of all the information about COVID-19 vaccines."

The survey also asked Americans for their reactions to changing public health guidance around some aspects of the pandemic, including information about how the virus spreads and how effective masks are in limiting its spread. Three-quarters or more of unvaccinated Americans expressed negative reactions to the changing guidance, such as by saying it made them wonder if public health officials were holding back important information (78%) and that it made them less confident in public health officials' recommendations (75%).

8.

Most vaccinated Americans—but not all—say they would probably get a booster shot if recommended by public health officials. The U.S. Food and Drug Administration recently approved an additional dose of a COVID-19 vaccine for Americans with weakened immune systems, and booster shots could be in the works for a broader swath of the public, too. In August, a large majority of vaccinated adults—amounting to 62% of all U.S. adults—said they would probably get a vaccine booster if recommended. But a small segment of vaccinated adults—amounting to 10% of all adults—said they would probably not get a booster shot.

9.

Americans have mixed views about vaccine requirements in public places. Majorities said in August that they favor requiring adults to show proof of COVID-19 vaccination to travel by airplane (61%), attend public colleges and universities in person (57%) and go to a sporting event or concert (56%). But the public was evenly divided over such a requirement for eating inside a restaurant (50% favored it, 50% opposed it), and slightly more likely to oppose than favor proof of vaccination for shopping inside stores and businesses (54% vs. 45%).

Americans' views on these questions were closely linked to party affiliation: Majorities of Democrats favored requiring proof of vaccination in each of these five settings, while majorities of Republicans were opposed in all five cases. Public attitudes were also tied to vaccination status, with majorities of vaccinated adults favoring proof of vaccination in all five settings and unvaccinated adults overwhelmingly opposed.

The public was also divided over how U.S. businesses should approach vaccinations. Around four-in-ten adults (39%) said most businesses should require employees to get a COVID-19 vaccine, while 35% say businesses should encourage but not require it. A quarter of adults said businesses should neither require nor encourage it. Here, too, views were linked to party affiliation and vaccination status. The survey was conducted before President Joe Biden announced that employers with more than 100 workers would be required to have their employees vaccinated or tested weekly for COVID-19.

10.

Few Americans know there is little access to COVID-19 vaccines in developing countries—and few say it should be a top priority for the U.S. to provide such nations with large numbers of vaccines. Only around a quarter of U.S. adults (26%) correctly said in August that very few people in developing countries have access to coronavirus vaccines.

On a separate question, 26% of adults said it should be a top priority for the U.S. to provide large numbers of COVID-19 vaccines to developing countries. Around half (49%) said it should be an important priority but not a top priority, while 23% said that it should be a lower priority or that it should not be done at all. Democrats were more than three times as likely as Republicans to say it should be a top priority for the U.S. to provide large numbers of vaccines to developing countries (39% vs. 11%); Republicans, in turn, were roughly four times as likely as Democrats to say it should be a lower priority or should not be done at all (40% vs. 9%).

Viewpoint 2

> *"The consensus among likely voters is that the federal government should do less, not more."*

Democratic Voters Favor Vaccinations Against COVID-19

Christopher Talgo, Justin Haskins, and Jim Lakely

In the following viewpoint Christopher Talgo, Justin Haskins, and Jim Lakely report on a poll that demonstrates how a person's political affiliation affects how they feel about the COVID-19 vaccine and how they would possibly treat unvaccinated individuals. Rasmussen Reports argues through presented statistics how deeply divided Americans are in their beliefs, which appear to correlate along political party lines. Rasmussen Reports is a media company specializing in the publication, collection, and distribution of public opinion information. Christopher Talgo, Justin Haskins, and Jim Lakely are affiliated with the Heartland Institute.

As you read, consider the following questions:

1. According to the report, which political party supports the Biden administration's vaccine mandate plan?
2. Which demographic supported fining or imprisoning doubters?

"Press Release: Heartland/Rasmussen Poll: Democrats Still Support Draconian COVID Measures", by Christopher Talgo, Justin Haskins, and Jim Lakely, Heartland Institute, January 12, 2022. Reprinted by permission.

3. Which political affiliation trusts the vaccine, according to the viewpoint?

Democrats are much more likely than those not in the party to support government restricting and tracking the movement of those who have not received the COVID-19 vaccine, silencing any speech that questions the efficacy of the vaccine, and punishing the unvaccinated with fines and imprisonment.

A new poll by The Heartland Institute and Rasmussen Reports found a deep partisan divide on COVID-19 policy in America. The survey of 1,016 likely voters, completed on January 5, 2022, found that 59% of Democrats support government forcing Americans to remain confined in their homes if they refuse the COVID vaccine. Only 17% of Republicans supported that idea with 79% opposed.

An overwhelming majority of Democrats (78%) support President Biden's vaccine mandate for private businesses with more than 100 employees, which stands before the U.S. Supreme Court. A majority of Democrats say Americans who don't get COVID-19 vaccines should be subject to fines (55%). Only 34% of all likely voters surveyed agreed.

A plurality of Democrats said governments should "fine or imprison individuals who publicly question the efficacy of the existing COVID-19 vaccines" (48%), and support forcing unvaccinated American citizens "to use a smart phone app or wearable device that tracks unvaccinated people to ensure that they are quarantined or socially distancing from others." Only 27% of likely voters overall agreed with punishing vaccine skeptics, and only 28% overall supported tracking the unvaccinated.

Though not near a majority, or even a plurality, the highest category of respondents who "strongly support" or "somewhat support" a proposal to "temporarily remove parents' custody of their children if parents refuse to take the COVID-19 vaccine" were Democrats (29%). Republicans opposed that idea 90% to 7%.

As for Dr. Anthony Fauci, who has controlled COVID-19 policy in America since the Trump administration, the poll of likely voters found an almost even split with 45% having either a very or somewhat favorable impression and 48% a somewhat or very unfavorable impression. However, three-fourths of Democrats and self-identified liberals approve of Dr. Fauci while more than two-thirds of Republicans and self-identified conservatives disapprove.

"After two excruciatingly long years, likely voters are beginning to question the federal government's handling of the pandemic," said Chris Talgo, senior editor and research fellow at The Heartland Institute, which commissioned this poll. "First and foremost, likely voters are beginning to sour on Dr. Anthony Fauci, who seems to have lost credibility after countless flip-flops.

A Summary of Democrats' Support of Draconian COVID Measures

Nearly two years after former President Donald Trump tossed politics into the nation's battle against the coronavirus, the partisan divide appears to have grown, with Republicans fighting mandates and Democrats calling for harsh punishments for those who refuse to get vaccinated.

In an expanded survey of the public's view of mandates and punishments to get people vaccinated, Rasmussen Reports found that Democrats even support fines, home confinement, and prison for those who fight the government on masks and shots.

Over several questions in the survey for the Heartland Institute, the differences in how Republicans and Democrats view the crisis were stark.

Consider: Twenty-nine percent of Democrats would go so far as to support taking children away from parents who refused to be vaccinated.

The first question in the survey set the tone. It asked if likely voters approved of coronavirus czar Dr. Anthony Fauci. Just 21% of Republicans said they view him favorably, compared to 75% of Democrats.

Next came a question on President Joe Biden's mandate that companies of 100 employees or more should demand workers to

"Moreover, almost half of likely voters oppose President Biden's vaccine mandates, which seem less about stopping the spread of COVID-19 and more about increasing the power of the federal government," Talgo said. "When asked about several other potential strategies, such as fining those who refuse to get vaccinated, the consensus among likely voters is that the federal government should do less, not more."

The Heartland Institute is a national nonprofit organization founded in 1984 and headquartered in Arlington Heights, Illinois. Its mission is to discover, develop, and promote free-market solutions to social and economic problems.

get vaccinated. Just 22% of Republicans agreed, while Democrats were all in at 78%.

Asked if voters favor a federal or state fine for those who refuse a vaccine, only 19% of Republicans said "favor" to 55% of Democrats.

Rasmussen next asked if people favor home confinement for those who are not vaccinated. On the GOP side, 79% were opposed, while 59% of Democrats favored it.

The survey also asked about those who challenge the government's view of vaccines and if opponents should be jailed or fined for questioning it on social media. A remarkable 48% of Democrats supported those punishments.

And nearly half of Democrats favored fixing tracking devices on those who refused to vaccinate.

Rasmussen added that Biden supporters would go even further than Democrats.

"President Biden's strongest supporters are most likely to endorse the harshest punishments against those who won't get the COVID-19 vaccine. Among voters who have a Very Favorable impression of Biden, 51% are in favor of government putting the unvaccinated in "designated facilities," and 54% favor imposing fines or prison sentences on vaccine critics," said the pollster.

"Democrats OK with Fines, Prison, and Mandates for Vaccine Deniers: Poll," by Paul Bedard, Washington Examiner, January 13, 2022.

National Survey of 1,016 Likely Voters on COVID-19 Policies

Conducted January 5, 2022

By The Heartland Institute and Rasmussen Reports

Do you have a very favorable, somewhat favorable, somewhat unfavorable or very unfavorable impression of Dr. Anthony Fauci?

28% - very favorable

17% - somewhat favorable

14% - somewhat unfavorable

34% - very unfavorable

8% - you are not sure

INTERESTING CROSSTAB: Some of Fauci's highest approval ratings came from Democrats (75%) and Blacks (58%), and more people between the ages of 18-39 (47%) approved of him than those over 65 (44%). Only 38% of Independents had a favorable impression of Fauci.

Do you strongly favor, somewhat favor, somewhat oppose or strongly oppose President Biden's plan to impose a COVID-19 vaccine mandate on the employees of large companies and government agencies?

33% - strongly favor

15% - somewhat favor

8% - somewhat oppose

40% - strongly oppose

4% - not sure

INTERESTING CROSSTAB: 58% of those between the ages of 18-39 strongly or somewhat support this policy, while fully half of people 40-64 strongly oppose it.

Would you strongly favor, somewhat favor, somewhat oppose or strongly oppose a proposal for federal or state governments to fine Americans who choose not to get a COVID-19 vaccine?

21% - strongly favor
13% - somewhat favor
14% - somewhat oppose
44% - strongly oppose
8% - not sure

INTERESTING CROSSTAB: 53% of self-identified liberals favor this policy, while 72% of conservatives oppose it. Older voters are strongly against while voters under 40 were most-likely to approve (45%).

Would you strongly favor, somewhat favor, somewhat oppose or strongly oppose a proposal to limit the spread of the coronavirus by having federal or state governments require that citizens remain confined to their homes at all times, except for emergencies, if they refuse to get a COVID-19 vaccine?

18% - strongly favor
16% - somewhat favor
14% - somewhat oppose
47% - strongly oppose
5% - not sure

INTERESTING CROSSTAB: Half of all Black voters and 58% of voters who identified themselves as liberals favored this policy. Nearly half (48%) of voters under 40 favored it.

Would you strongly favor, somewhat favor, somewhat oppose or strongly oppose a proposal to limit the spread of the coronavirus by having federal or state governments require that citizens temporarily live in designated facilities or locations if they refuse to get a COVID-19 vaccine?

13% - strongly favor
13% - somewhat favor
13% - somewhat oppose
58% - strongly oppose
3% - not sure

INTERESTING CROSSTAB: The breakdown of "strongly oppose" was conservatives (78%), moderates (71%), and liberals (36%).

Would you strongly favor, somewhat favor, somewhat oppose or strongly oppose a proposal for federal or state governments to fine or imprison individuals who publicly question the efficacy of the existing COVID-19 vaccines on social media, television, radio, or in online or digital publications?

13% - strongly favor

14% - somewhat favor

14% - somewhat oppose

53% - strongly oppose

6% - not sure

INTERESTING CROSSTAB: Younger voters between the ages of 18-40 were the most likely to support fining or imprisoning those who express doubts about the COVID vaccines (39%).

Would you strongly favor, somewhat favor, somewhat oppose or strongly oppose a proposal for federal or state governments to require unvaccinated citizens to use a smart phone app or wearable device that tracks unvaccinated people to ensure that they are quarantined or socially distancing from others?

13% - strongly favor

15% - somewhat favor

11% - somewhat oppose

55% - strongly oppose

5% - not sure

INTERESTING CROSSTAB: More than half of younger voters (53%) support government tracking apps. A strong majority of moderates (70%) were opposed.

Would you strongly favor, somewhat favor, somewhat oppose or strongly oppose a proposal to temporarily remove parents' custody of their children if parents refuse to take the COVID-19 vaccine?

9% - strongly favor

7% - somewhat favor

13% - somewhat oppose

67% - strongly oppose

4% - not sure

INTERESTING CROSSTAB: This was a very unpopular policy idea, but the largest demographics in support of government removing children from unvaccinated parents were voters between the ages of 18-39 (31%), Democrats (29%), and liberals, Blacks, and Hispanics (24%). Only 13% of white voters favored it.

NOTE: Margin of Sampling Error, +/- 3 percentage points with a 95% level of confidence

Viewpoint 3

> *"...many Republican men interviewed...said they were concerned about side effects, or said they distrusted federal health agencies and the government."*

Republican Men Are Vaccine-Hesitant, but There's Little Focus on Them

Aallyah Wright

In the following viewpoint Aallyah Wright outlines vaccine hesitancy and zeroes in to concentrate on men who self-identify as Republicans. Wright maintains that many in this group distrust vaccines for one reason or another. Wright highlights several Republican men who argue for getting a COVID vaccine, and some that get the vaccine without endorsing it publicly. Wright also presents the views of several doctors, both for and against the COVID vaccine. Aallyah Wright reports on rural affairs, race, and equity issues for Stateline, a daily and weekly newsletter for Pew Charitable Trusts.

As you read, consider the following questions:

1. Which group of Republican men has the largest share of vaccine hesitancy according to Wright?
2. Are all Republican men adverse to vaccines?

"Republican Men Are Vaccine-Hesitant, but There's Little Focus on Them," by Aallyah Wright, The Pew Charitable Trusts, April 23, 2021. Copyright ©The Pew Charitable Trusts. All Rights Reserved. Reproduced with permission. Any use without the express written consent of The Pew Charitable Trusts is prohibited.

3. How can vaccine hesitancy be overcome?

In December, Arizona Republican state Rep. Mark Finchem suffered from flu-like symptoms—headache, fatigue, body aches and chills. But it wasn't the flu; he tested positive for COVID-19. Nearly three months later, his mother, who had recently contracted the coronavirus, died after battling throat cancer for over 40 years.

Those circumstances weren't enough to persuade Finchem, who is in his early 60s, to get a Moderna, Pfizer-BioNTech or Johnson & Johnson COVID-19 vaccine. Finchem remains skeptical, he said, because he distrusts the federal government and top public health officials, he's heard mixed messages about the vaccines on social media and television news, and he worries about long-term side effects.

"I'm very suspicious that what they put in the [vaccines] is nothing more than a cocktail," Finchem said in a phone call with Stateline. "Time will tell, and I hope I'm proven wrong."

As federal and state government entities ramp up vaccination efforts, polls show increased confidence in vaccines, especially among people of color, who have been disproportionately affected by COVID-19 and were, at least initially, more skeptical of the vaccines. Vaccine hesitancy persists across all demographics, however.

About 13% of American adults don't want a COVID-19 vaccine, according to the Kaiser Family Foundation. Republicans are the most resistant; nearly 3 in 10 say they don't want one. The share is greater among rural, Republican men, 35% of whom don't want to get a vaccine.

So far, more than 200 million complete doses of COVID-19 have been administered in the United States, which amounts to about 34% of U.S. adults being fully vaccinated. The percentage of vaccinated adults needed to reach herd immunity is widely debated, but many scientists say the country must top 80% of the adult population. And to achieve that goal, public health officials say, it is important to alleviate concerns among all people.

To that end, many state and county health departments have made special efforts to reach Black, Hispanic, homebound and unhoused populations that have been hit hard by the pandemic. By contrast, few, if any, have mounted Republican-specific initiatives to combat hesitancy.

There are a variety of reasons why people decline to be vaccinated, said Howard Gamble, administrator for the Wheeling-Ohio County Health Department in West Virginia. Gamble recalled a father who recently brought his 17-year-old daughter to get vaccinated. When Gamble asked the father whether he also wanted his first dose, the man's response was, "I just don't do these kinds of things." Persistent misinformation on social media about the coronavirus and vaccines can drive people from getting inoculated, Gamble said.

"It's not very simplistic or cut and dry," Gamble said. "We see a lot of reasons."

Like Finchem, the Arizona lawmaker, many Republican men interviewed by Stateline said they were concerned about side effects, or said they distrusted federal health agencies and the government. Finchem, like most Republicans, doesn't believe that President Joe Biden's victory in the November election was legitimate, for example. Some of the GOP men said vaccine manufacturers were just interested in making money.

And many of them are in positions of leadership and influence.

For North Dakota Republican state Rep. Rick Becker, hesitancy isn't the reason for his hang-ups about vaccines, he said. Becker, a plastic surgeon, said he doesn't plan to be vaccinated because he knows he is healthy and that there is only a small chance that the coronavirus would kill him. Becker, 56, says he does not have any preexisting health conditions and thinks his choice will not affect others.

"People should be making up their own minds," he said. "If a person is choosing to look at elected officials, they're not afforded the proper diligence of their own decision. You do what's best for you."

State Rep. Brady Williamson, a 44-year-old Republican from Mississippi, said he's unsure whether he'll get a vaccine because it hasn't been out for a long time. He also argued that he doesn't need it because he is "in the gym and fit" and doesn't have underlying health conditions. He said he doesn't like the government to make decisions for individuals, businesses and churches.

Not all Republican men are so staunchly resistant.

At 70 years old, longtime Georgia state Rep. Tommy Benton said it would be foolish for him and others in his age group to turn down a vaccine. Benton, who doesn't have underlying health conditions, didn't want to catch COVID-19 or transmit it to his grandkids or peers, he said.

"It doesn't matter how healthy you are. At…65 or above, you might end up getting sick with this disease and it'll be more than your 65-or-above system can handle," Benton said.

Wyoming state Rep. Daniel Zwonitzer, 41, who lives in the most vaccine-hesitant state in the country, said he took a vaccine for the safety of others, particularly for the older staff, legislators and volunteers in the Wyoming legislature. While Zwonitzer believes in freedom and liberty, he said, he also believes in public health. Zwonitzer does not have any preexisting health conditions, he noted.

He said a few of his Republican colleagues think COVID-19 and vaccines against it are a hoax, but he disagreed, pointing out that one of his fellow Republicans died from the disease.

Some Republican men and health officials cited the politicization of mask-wearing and shutdowns under former President Donald Trump's administration, and its downplaying of the seriousness of the pandemic, as causes for the vaccine hesitancy among conservatives.

Early last year, the Trump administration made false claims that the coronavirus had been contained and COVID-19 infections were declining, despite statistics showing rising numbers.

The counties that are most vaccine-hesitant are rural, more likely to support Trump and have lower income levels and college graduation rates, The New York Times recently reported. In these rural, more Republican-leaning areas, health officials said, vaccine supply often exceeds demand.

Debra Furr-Holden, an epidemiologist at Michigan State University's School of Public Health, said many Republican men have taken cues from party leaders, who spent months last year downplaying the pandemic's effects.

"They were COVID deniers when the pandemic first started and aren't willing to admit, 'Hey, we were wrong,'" Furr-Holden said. "They're thinking, 'So if it was no big deal, why should getting the vaccine be a big deal?'"

Some top Republican leaders, meanwhile, have more recently urged those who are hesitant to take the vaccines.

"I can say as a Republican man, as soon as it was my turn, I took the vaccine," Senate Minority Leader Mitch McConnell said at a news conference in March. "I would encourage all Republican men to do that."

Trump did get vaccinated, quietly and not in front of cameras, shortly before leaving office in January. Last month, in a Fox News interview, he urged unvaccinated Americans to get shots. "I would recommend it, and I would recommend it to a lot of people that don't want to get it, and a lot of those people voted for me, frankly," he said.

"We have our freedoms and we have to live by that, and I agree with that also," he said. "But it is a great vaccine. It is a safe vaccine and it is something that works."

But nearly 80% of Republicans said Trump's endorsement would not make them more likely to get a vaccine, according to a recent poll by the Kaiser Family Foundation. The Republican men Stateline interviewed said Trump's support of the vaccine did not sway their decisions.

Republican state Sen. Ralph Alvarado of Kentucky, a 50-year-old physician, said instead of shaming people who are reluctant to get vaccinated, it's crucial to understand their concerns. He said he spends a lot of time dispelling myths about vaccines among his constituents, patients and community.

"As a doctor, I remind my colleagues that when we prescribe or recommend a course of action for somebody, no matter what the disease or prevention is, if people become resistant or hesitant, our medical code of ethics doesn't say to humiliate," he said. "You reassure and educate them."

He added that a lot of people are fearful when politics is involved, because "people pick sides instead of picking the message."

Public health experts also have stressed the need to focus outreach efforts on science. An analysis published in Health Affairs, a peer-reviewed health journal, stated that when "science and values, not politics, inform public health," it "unlocks potential for higher vaccine coverage."

Daniel Salmon, one of the report's authors and director of the Institute for Vaccine Safety at the Johns Hopkins Bloomberg School of Public Health, elaborated in an interview. Instead of trying to persuade people to get vaccinated, he said, public health officials should sit down with community members and tell them, "'This is what we know, and this is what we don't know, and this is what we're doing to figure out what we don't know.' It has to come from trusted leaders. It has to be well-informed. That's the way it's done, one community at a time."

The de Beaumont Foundation, a Maryland-based charitable foundation focused on health solutions, held a two-hour session with a focus group in March that found messaging helps to build trust. The group consisted of almost 20 people who identified as conservative Republicans who supported Trump.

"We found that we're able to [increase vaccine confidence] by really delivering the facts and giving people the freedom to make the choice," Brian Castrucci, an epidemiologist and president and CEO of the de Beaumont Foundation, told Stateline. "You can read the facts all day, but if they seem to perceive you are trying to manipulate their decision or if you're threatening their freedom, walls go up that aren't easily undone."

The Casper-Natrona County Health Department in Wyoming learned through surveys that accessibility, technology and education issues hindered some people from getting shots. After hearing from Republican men, Bloom said, officials learned that many were concerned about vaccine technology and how it works.

The Spokane, Washington, office of the federal Department of Veterans Affairs also is tailoring its approach to community concerns. It currently drives a mobile unit through rural Washington, Idaho and Montana to deliver vaccinations to rural veterans, many of whom are Republican men, even though most veterans contacted by the office have said they don't want the shots, according to The Washington Post.

The Michigan Department of Health and Human Services plans to get more Republicans and conservatives vaccinated by partnering with trusted leaders, expanding its mobile vaccinations and hosting virtual community town halls to answer questions about vaccine safety and effectiveness, reported Bridge Michigan.

At the national level, the U.S. Department of Health and Human Services announced the "We Can Do It" campaign to combat vaccine hesitancy. The Ad Council and COVID Collaborative rolled out an education campaign specifically for religious groups and conservative Americans. The campaign focuses on how clinical trials were conducted, the science of the development, and support of COVID-19 vaccines by doctors.

The initiative uses social media, celebrity influencers, advertisements and partnerships with rural, medical and faith-based organizations to reach these groups.

Castrucci praised the work of the Ad Council, but said it needs to be complemented by an on-the-ground perspective from local pastors, doctors and families.

"Concern should be normalized. At the end of the day, everyone wants information. … We have to make sure the messaging works for the people that are getting the messages."

Viewpoint 4

"...the political right and the anti-vaccine movement are drawing ever-closer together. It's an alliance that promises to give both sides more power, but the cost is potentially thousands of American lives."

Pro-Trump Republicans Struck an Alliance with Anti-Vaccine Activists

Geoff Brumfiel

In the following viewpoint Geoff Brumfiel demonstrates that the joining of two factions, the anti-vaxxers and the political right, is a potent, dangerous mix of ideologies. Brumfiel outlines the joining of these two forces in America and presents a case of how disturbing this mix can be for both politics and public health. Brumfiel provides evidence that shows how personalities in both political and anti-vaccine ideology are pushing their agendas to win converts to their way of thinking. Geoff Brumfiel is a senior editor and correspondent for NPR's science desk.

As you read, consider the following questions:

1. According to the viewpoint, are all anti-vaxxers Republican?
2. Are politicians joining with anti-vaxx supporters for political reasons or public health reasons?
3. Who is pummeling Republican voters with bad science?

©2021 National Public Radio, Inc. NPR news report titled "Inside the growing alliance between anti-vaccine activists and pro-Trump Republicans" by Geoff Brumfiel was originally published on npr.org on December 6, 2021, and is used with the permission of NPR. Any unauthorized duplication is strictly prohibited.

In October, a conference filled with anti-vaccine activists in Nashville, Tenn., received a high-profile political guest: former President Donald Trump's son Eric Trump.

While portions of the younger Trump's half-hour address were typical political platitudes, some of his biggest applause lines came when he attacked COVID-19 vaccine mandates.

"Do you want to get a vaccine or do you not? Do you want to be left alone or not?" said Trump to a roaring audience.

Still, Trump's emphasis was very different from those of many of the other speakers at the event, put on by longtime anti-vaccine activists Ty and Charlene Bollinger.

The day before Trump's speech, a homeopathic doctor named Edward Group stood on the same stage and suggested to the audience they should drink their urine as an alternative to getting vaccinated against COVID-19. Another speaker, Carrie Madej, said the vaccines contained microscopic technology designed to put "another kind of nervous system inside you." The true purpose of the vaccines, she claimed, was to turn humans into cyborgs.

It's the sort of fringe views that kept political figures away from this conference in the past. But as America heads into midterm elections next year, the political right and the anti-vaccine movement are drawing ever-closer together. It's an alliance that promises to give both sides more power, but the cost is potentially thousands of American lives.

To understand what's going on, it's important to understand where the parties are coming from. The anti-vaccine movement was not always especially political. Some of the movement's leaders, such as Robert F. Kennedy Jr., the son of the late Democratic Sen. Robert F. Kennedy, have championed other liberal causes in the past.

An Outrageous and Irresponsible Claim from a U.S. Senator

Brianna Keilar was disturbed about the latest vaccine conspiracy theory touted by GOPer Ron Johnson, quite possibly the dumbest man in the Senate:

"We've heard story after story. I mean, all these athletes dropping dead on the field. But we're supposed to ignore that. Nothing happening here. Nothing to see. This is a travesty. This is a scandal."

And here to fact-check this strange new COVID conspiracy theory is reporter and editor-at-large Chris Cillizza.

"In December, Gateway Pundit, which is a very pro-Trump website that publishes lots of things that aren't true, linked to a study from a site called Good Sciencing, which said, oh, well, there's all these athletes with myocarditis and pericarditis. The problem is, it's just not accurate. Some of the people they said are Hank Aaron, who at 86 died in 2021. It was from natural causes, according to the Fulton County medical examiner. They named a Danish soccer player who had a heart attack during the Euro competition last year but had not been vaccinated. So it doesn't take a lot of digging. It barely takes any digging at all to find out that this stuff just isn't true," Cillizza said.

"The idea that Ron Johnson would give it a forum with, you know, his stature as a United States senator, it should be shocking. It isn't, given his track record. It is still appalling, in my opinion."

How much digging does it take to know that Gateway Pundit is so riddled with untruths, it was permanently kicked off Twitter a year ago? Or that Jim Hoft, its founder, has the honorary title of Dumbest Man On The Internet?

How hard would it have been for the reporter who was interviewing Johnson to ask those questions?

"Ron Johnson Claims 150 Athletes Dropped Dead From Vaccine," by Susie Madrak, Crooks and Liars, January 28, 2022.

An Unlikely Alliance

"The truth is, I'm still a registered Democrat," says Del Bigtree, a well-known anti-vaccine activist. Even before COVID-19, he wrote and produced a documentary that falsely claimed childhood vaccines were linked to autism. But the message never caught on with the liberal audience he was targeting.

Instead, it seemed to tap into something on the political right. He still remembers the first time he noticed; it was after he was invited to speak at a conservative women's group in Texas.

"Clearly I was shocked as a lifelong liberal progressive that I was hugging and hanging out and having a great time with a bunch of extremely conservative mothers and grandmothers," says Bigtree.

Bigtree has been banned from social media platforms like YouTube for making false claims about the dangers of COVID-19 vaccines. But as the pandemic has dragged on, his conservative audience keeps growing. Often he speaks at conferences alongside people who claim the election was rigged and promoters of QAnon conspiracy theories.

"Unless there's going to be a white supremacist on the stage or I find out that there's something that I truly find distasteful, then I just see that stage as simply an audience that I want to hear this message," says Bigtree.

It's a numbers game. He wants to grow his movement, and he'll talk to anyone who will listen.

On the other side of this alliance are far-right conservatives like Trump's former political adviser Roger Stone. Stone has been a Republican political operative since the 1970s, beginning with Richard Nixon's 1972 campaign. He's a longtime friend of Trump's and was convicted of lying to Congress about his knowledge of the 2016 Trump campaign's contacts with Russia. Trump pardoned Stone in December 2020.

Stone, who spoke at the conference, says he's quite open to some of the ideas presented there about vaccines. But he also sees the shot as a powerful wedge issue that Republicans can use to motivate conservative voters during next year's midterm elections. Citing public polls, Stone says that in particular, vaccine mandates are "highly likely" to be a campaign issue.

Vaccine mandates have many features that make them a good issue to motivate conservative voters. It invokes a fight about the government regulation and personal liberty. But add in the apocalyptic views of anti-vaccine activists and the political power of arguments against vaccine mandates gets punched up to a whole new level.

For example, Bigtree falsely claims that the COVID-19 vaccines are killing people and represent an existential threat to humanity: "I believe that this vaccine approach, this vaccine itself, this brand-new technology, is so incredibly dangerous, that we are actually putting our species at risk."

It's the synergy between real politics and imagined dangers that is bringing the pro-Trump movement and anti-vaccine activists together.

But the result of this union increasingly appears to be an even higher death toll from COVID-19, in part because it's causing many people to resist getting the shot.

"We find a huge correlation between belief in misinformation and being unvaccinated," says Liz Hamel, who heads public opinion research with the Kaiser Family Foundation, a nonpartisan health care think tank.

Between conservative media and GOP politicians, many Republican voters are being pummeled with bad science about vaccines almost daily. Kaiser's polling found that 94% of Republicans think one or more false statements about COVID-19 and vaccine safety might be true.

Over the past eight months, Hamel has watched as Republican vaccination rates have fallen further and further behind the rest of America. While Republicans tracked with other groups in terms of vaccination rates earlier this year, Kaiser's research shows that now, an unvaccinated person is three times as likely to lean Republican as they are to lean Democrat.

COVID Now Affecting Republicans More

A new analysis by NPR suggests that Republicans are probably dying at a higher rate as a result. A nationwide comparison of 2020 presidential election results and COVID-19 death rates since vaccines became available for all adults, found that counties that voted heavily for Trump had nearly three times the COVID-19 mortality rate of those that went for Joe Biden. Those counties also had far lower vaccination rates.

The analysis only provides a geographic association, and the individual political affiliations of those taken by COVID-19 remains unknown. "It's a little crass to ask someone what their loved one's ideology was after they passed away," says Charles Gaba, an independent health care analyst who has been tracking partisanship trends during the pandemic. But the strength of the association, combined with polling information, strongly suggests that Republicans are being disproportionately affected.

When asked about Republicans' low vaccination rates, Stone was nonplussed. "Each person must make their own choice, God bless them." He went on to falsely claim that getting the vaccine actually enhances a person's chance of getting the disease. "So I guess I'd be more concerned if I were a Democrat," he says.

Other conservative politicians try to avoid the thorny issue by keeping the conversation on the issue of choice. "It's not about whether the vaccines work or not," says Mark Burns, a conservative pastor closely affiliated with Donald Trump. "What matters for me is that you are stripping citizens [of] the right to choose what's best for their own life."

Burns, who is running for Congress in South Carolina, likened the choice about vaccination to smoking: "Cigarettes kill people every day, but yet you can go to the supermarket right now and buy it with no issue, that's their choice. If they want to go put cancer into their lungs, they have a right to do so." He felt his position would help him win the primary in the conservative district where he hopes to be elected.

"The Worst Element in American Politics Today"

But for many Republicans who are concerned about public health, the willingness to parlay a lifesaving vaccine into political capital is disturbing.

"They just care about winning," says Annette Meeks, a lifelong Republican who heads the Freedom Foundation of Minnesota conservative think tank. "It's the worst element in American politics today."

Meeks has seen the data on vaccines, and she's watched people she knows get sick. "To see people reject those vaccines based on pseudoscience or worse—lies—and to see lives lost is a tragedy beyond words," Meeks says.

In addition to the moral failings, Meeks says embracing the anti-vaccine movement carries huge political risks for the GOP. That's because elections in states like Minnesota are won and lost in the suburbs. And those suburban voters tend to be vaccinated.

"I believe that the long-term consequences for the Republican Party will be a lot of those independent suburban voters will look askance at us and say, 'What is this all about? I got vaccinated, my whole family got vaccinated, and we're just fine.'"

The risks for the Republican Party in lives and votes may be real, but the there is little downside for the other party in this alliance—the anti-vaccine movement.

Del Bigtree says he's seeing more people at speaking engagements and getting millions of visitors to his website each week.

"We are growing in size, in numbers, in confidence and in finances," he says. And for now, his audience is clear: conservative America.

Viewpoint 5

> *"...on the frontline of these anti-vax protests are people occupied by extreme rage who are threatening to exert violence against whoever they deem as 'outsiders' and 'traitors.'"*

Anti-Vaccine Beliefs and Actions Increase with Political Extremism

Sibo Chen

In the following viewpoint Sibo Chen draws a distinction between historically significant vaccine hesitancy and what is seen today as a far-right induced hesitancy. Chen argues that political extremism has infiltrated the ranks of the anti-vaccine establishment, and consequently, members of this group may be acting more violent. Chen maintains that very specific reasons are to blame for this heightened extreme anti-vaccine movement. Sibo Chen is an assistant professor at Ryerson University, and an expert in risk and crisis communication.

As you read, consider the following questions:

1. Historically, what are the three reasons for vaccine hesitancy?
2. What is a present-day reason for vaccine hesitancy according to the author?
3. How is the public sphere broken as stated by the viewpoint?

"The Anti-Vax Movement Is Being Radicalized by Far-Right Political Extremism," by Sibo Chen, The Conversation, September 19, 2021. https://theconversation.com/the-anti-vax-movement-is-being-radicalized-by-far-right-political-extremism-166396. Licensed under CC BY-ND 4.0 International.

Vaccine passports have become a major point of contention in the 2021 federal election.

Currently, more than 73 per cent of Canada's population have received at least one dose of vaccine, and the country's response to COVID-19 continues to be a top priority for voters. This is likely why current public health efforts have concentrated on expanding vaccine access and implementing communication strategies (like motivational interviewing) to increase vaccination rates.

But, as seen through recent anti-vax protests, especially those targeting schools and hospitals, there is a worrisome convergence of the anti-vaccine movement and far-right political extremism.

And on the frontline of these anti-vax protests are people occupied by extreme rage who are threatening to exert violence against whoever they deem as "outsiders" and "traitors."

For decades, vaccine hesitancy has been a subject of intense study in the field of scientific communication. The issue's recent radicalization makes insights about its root causes even more important.

Factors Contributing to Vaccine Hesitancy

A distinction must be drawn between vaccine hesitancy and the current anti-vax movement, as the latter's agenda has been hijacked by far-right groups.

Previous study has identified a variety of factors contributing to people's vaccination hesitancy, such as community trauma, scientific scepticism and political beliefs. Some Indigenous communities' concerns about COVID-19 vaccines, for instance, come from instances of medical experimentation.

Meanwhile, errors made during pro-vaccine communications may raise additional concerns about vaccination safety and efficacy. Consider the public uncertainty and outrage over the National Advisory Committee on Immunization's contradictory messages regarding AstraZeneca.

Research on vaccine hesitancy around the world has demonstrated that a number of contributing factors to vaccine hesitation are directly linked to a persistent decline in public trust in institutions and government policy. In recent years, this trend, along with escalating political polarization, has shaped the anti-vaccine movement into its current form.

Prior to the pandemic, researchers noted that social media platforms, like Facebook, facilitate anti-vaccine messages and conspiracy theories by enabling the diffusion of misinformation like "pesticides caused clinical symptoms of polio." Fast forwarding to 2020, major anti-vaccine groups on Facebook launched anti-vaccine misinformation campaigns weeks before the U.S. government launched its vaccine development program, sewing seeds of doubt and subsequently hampering the rollout of COVID-19 vaccines across the country.

The Radicalization of the Anti-Vaccine Movement

Since the start of mass COVID-19 vaccinations in [late] 2020, the public health sector has been closely monitoring an unusually high level of resistance among a small section of the population. Unlike prior vaccination hesitancy, the current anti-vax movement cannot be explained by a lack of information or illogical thinking, especially in light of the significant press coverage and public health initiatives over the last several months.

Scholars have resorted to the solution aversion model to account for the growing political division around vaccination. According to this model, individuals with divergent political ideologies perceive social issues differently because of their inherent aversion to specific solutions. In the case of vaccine passports, its implementation depends on stringent government regulations, which are deeply unpopular among many far-right individuals.

Additionally, our fragmented media environment further fosters solution aversion by promoting motivated reasoning. With today's media audiences being trapped in algorithm-based digital echo chambers, it is increasingly typical for individuals to interact exclusively with like-minded media sources and other internet users, resulting in biased information absorption.

Fixing the Broken Public Sphere

Admittedly, reconciling the divided public opinions on COVID-19 vaccination policies is not a simple task. As long as social media platforms continue to not bat an eye at misinformation out of concern for their click-through rates, and governments continue to ignore structural injustices driving political radicalization, it is unlikely that vaccine resistance will be reduced without increasing polarization.

The anti-vax movement, like many other issues that have emerged during the pandemic, serves as a stark reminder that our society's public sphere is fundamentally broken. The long yet essential process of fixing it will require all of us, as responsible citizens and media users, to work collaboratively on restoring public conversation mechanisms.

Viewpoint 6

> *"Intelligence agencies around the world have warned of state-linked cyber operations targeting vaccines and vaccine manufacturers."*

Vaccine Mistrust and Disinformation Has Gone Global

Elise Thomas

In the following viewpoint Elise Thomas demonstrates how misinformation is spread on social media sites. Thomas demonstrates how this occurs, by using an example of a fictious press release and how it became part of a disinformation campaign on Twitter and Facebook. Thomas further demonstrates how the disinformation strategy spread, even though Facebook tried to dismantle the viral spread of misinformation. Elise Thomas is a researcher at the cyber policy center for Australian Strategic Policy Institute (ASPI).

As you read, consider the following questions:

1. As reported by the viewpoint, which two countries were targeted by the disinformation?
2. What evidence shows that Facebook was too late in taking down the story?
3. What is decontextualization as explained by the author?

"Covid-19 Disinformation Campaigns Shift Focus to Vaccines," by Elise Thomas, Australian Strategic Policy Institute, August 24, 2020. Reprinted by permission.

In ASPI's latest report on Covid-19 disinformation, Albert Zhang, Emilia Currey and I investigated how the narrative of an American vaccine trial killing soldiers in Ukraine (which did not actually happen) was laundered from the propaganda site of a pro-Russian militia into the international information ecosystem. What this case study highlights is the way in which the battle for control of the coronavirus narrative is shifting from the origins of the virus to the hopes for a vaccine.

On 17 July, a press release was posted in Russian and English on the website of the Lugansk People's Republic, a pro-Russian militia and self-declared government in Eastern Ukraine. The statement described a vaccine trial by "Americal [sic] virologists" in the Ukrainian-controlled city of Kharkiv which had led to the death of several volunteers, including Ukrainian soldiers.

From the beginning, this narrative had strong political undertones of both anti-Americanism and opposition to the legitimate Ukrainian government. The implication was that Americans did not value Ukrainian lives, and so wanted to test their dangerous vaccine on Ukrainians rather than on their own people—and that the puppet government in Kiev was letting them do it.

The completely fictional story was quickly picked up by Russian-language media and by a handful of fringe English-language conspiracy sites. Despite multiple fact-checks which found that no such incident ever occurred, the narrative swiftly established a foothold in the digital information ecosystem. Beginning with Russian-language outlet News.ru, the story was further embellished by attributing the deadly vaccine trial to US company Moderna and its mRNA-1273 vaccine candidate.

Intentionally or not, the effect of this move was to expand the appeal of the disinformation narrative to conspiracy and anti-vaxx communities. These communities' generic opposition to vaccinations has coalesced in recent weeks into a specific fixation on mRNA vaccines, which they believe change a person's DNA (they do not), among other things.

Our research has found that the disinformation narrative gained relatively little traction on English-language social media until 24 July, a week after it was originally published. On that day, Twitter and Facebook shares of English-language articles about the fictional vaccine trial suddenly and dramatically spiked.

This spike may be linked to an unusual viral Facebook post which began to spread that day, which is discussed in more detail in the report. It's difficult to reconstruct exactly what occurred, however, as Facebook appears to have clamped down on the viral growth of this piece of disinformation, deleting much of the relevant data in the process.

The clampdown came too late. Despite the best efforts of fact-checkers, the disinformation narrative of a US vaccine killing Ukrainian soldiers spread in multiple languages in addition to Russian and English, including Spanish, Italian, Romanian, Czech and French.

As of early August, it had effectively reached the final stage of the information-laundering cycle: decontextualisation. This is the phase in which the disinformation is just out there in the information ecosystem and asserted as fact, completely independent of its original context. It has since been incorporated into a range of other mis- and disinformation narratives, from conspiracies about US bioweapons labs in Ukraine to fuelling resistance to the Moderna vaccine in Canada.

This case study is one example of a broader shift which is taking place in the fight for control over the narrative around Covid-19. Earlier in the crisis, when there was a much greater international focus on the nature and origin of the virus, disinformation efforts were centred around those questions. We saw, for example, the duelling conspiracy theories about whether the virus escaped from a Wuhan lab or was created in a US Army medical facility and released in China.

As the global conversation shifts to the hopes for a vaccine, naturally the targets of disinformation efforts shift too. While the medical efficacy of any vaccine is essential, there's another ingredient which is crucial for the success of any mass vaccination effort: public trust.

Intelligence agencies around the world have warned of state-linked cyber operations targeting vaccines and vaccine manufacturers. Such efforts are aimed at stealing intellectual property to give a nation's vaccine candidates a leg-up in the race for the first safe and effective Covid-19 vaccine.

It should be assumed that some state and non-state actors are prepared to consider other tactics to give their own vaccine candidates the edge, including grey-zone disinformation campaigns. It's perhaps worth noting that the US–Ukraine vaccine disinformation was launched the day after Russia announced plans to mass-produce its own vaccine in a matter of weeks.

While it might have been hoped that the global search for a vaccine would be above this kind of geopolitical jostling, clearly that's not the case. Policymakers, media outlets, social media platforms and vaccine manufacturers should be aware that politically motivated disinformation is only likely to increase as the race for a Covid-19 vaccine intensifies.

Viewpoint 7

> *"The use of [vaccine] exemptions, particularly by parents on behalf of their school children, has been growing over the past decade."*

Religious Exemption to Circumvent Vaccination Has Increased

Associated Press

In the following viewpoint the Associated Press maintains that religious exemptions requested to circumvent vaccination while historically always used to some degree, have recently increased in the past decade. The author provides statistics showing vaccination rates of certain religious denominations while reporting on various ways people are using religion to refuse vaccinations and also details how certain employers and businesses are trying to ferret out sincere religious dissenters from those just not wanting a vaccine. The Associated Press is a nonprofit news agency.

As you read, consider the following questions:

1. According to the author, which federal law legislates over sincere religious beliefs?
2. Which major religious denomination quotes their leaders as saying it is "morally acceptable" to get a COVID-19 vaccination?
3. How has one Arkansas hospital tried to deal with religiously motivated vaccine refusal?

"As Covid-19 Vaccine Mandates Rise, Religious Exemptions Grow," Associated Press, September 16, 2021. Reprinted by permission.

About 3,000 Los Angeles Police Department employees are citing religious objections to try and get out of required Covid-19 vaccinations. In Washington State, thousands of State workers are seeking similar exemptions.

And an Arkansas hospital has been swamped with so many such requests from employees that it is apparently calling their bluff.

Religious objections, once used sparingly around the country to get exempted from various required vaccines, are becoming a much more widely used loophole against the Covid-19 shot.

And it is only likely to grow following President Joe Biden's sweeping new vaccine mandates covering more than 100 million Americans, including executive branch employees and workers at businesses with more than 100 people on the payroll.

The administration acknowledges that a small minority of Americans will use—and some may seek to exploit—religious exemptions. But it said it believes even marginal improvements in vaccination rates will save lives.

It is not clear how many federal employees have asked for a religious exemption, though union officials say there will be many requests. The Labor Department has said an accommodation can be denied if it causes an undue burden on the employer.

Various Exemptions

In the US, mask and vaccine requirements vary, but most offer exemptions for certain medical conditions or religious or philosophical objections. The use of such exemptions, particularly by parents on behalf of their school children, has been growing over the past decade.

The allowance was enshrined in the federal Civil Rights Act of 1964, which says employers must make reasonable accommodations for employees who object to work requirements because of "sincerely held" religious beliefs.

A religious belief does not have to be recognized by an organised religion, and it can be new, unusual or "seem illogical or unreasonable to others," according to rules laid out by the Equal Employment Opportunity Commission. But it can't be founded solely on political or social ideas.

That puts employers in the position of determining what is a legitimate religious belief and what is a dodge.

Controversial Vaccine

Many major religious denominations have no objections to the Covid-19 vaccines. But the rollout has prompted heated debates because of the long-time role that cell lines derived from fetal tissue have played, directly or indirectly, in the research and development of various vaccines and medicines.

Roman Catholic leaders in New Orleans and St. Louis went so far as to call Johnson & Johnson's Covid-19 shot "morally compromised." J&J has stressed that there is no fetal tissue in its vaccine.

Moreover, the Vatican's doctrine office has said it is "morally acceptable" for Catholics to receive Covid-19 vaccines that are based on research that used cells derived from aborted fetuses. Pope Francis himself has said it would be "suicide" not to get the shot, and he has been fully vaccinated with the Pfizer formula.

Religious Objections

In New York, State lawmakers have attempted to make the vaccine mandatory for medical workers, with no religious exemptions. On Tuesday, a federal judge blocked the State from enforcing the rule to give a group of workers time to argue that it is illegal because it lacks the opt-out.

An August AP-NORC poll found that 58 per cent of white evangelical Protestants, 72 per cent of white mainline Protestants, 80 per cent of Catholics and 73 per cent of Americans who are religiously unaffiliated say they have been vaccinated. Seventy percent of non-white Protestants say they have been, including 70 per cent of black Protestants.

Across the US, public officials, doctors and community leaders have been trying to help people circumvent Covid-19 mask and vaccine requirements.

In Tulsa, Oklahoma, pastor Jackson Lahmeyer is offering a "religious exemption" form on his church's website for download, along with links for suggested donations to the church. The 29-year-old is running for the US Senate as a Republican.

Anyone interested can get the form signed by a religious leader, or Lahmeyer can sign it himself if the person joins the church and donates. He said more than 35,000 people downloaded the form in just three days.

"We're not anti-vaxxers. We're just pro-freedom," Lahmeyer said. "A lot of these people who have signed ... have already taken the vaccine. They just don't think it's right that somebody else should be forced or lose their job."

But obtaining a religious exemption is not as simple as producing a signed form. Measles outbreaks in schools over the past decade prompted some States to change their policies. Some now require an actual signed affidavit from a religious leader, instead of an online form. California got rid of non-medical exemptions in 2015.

Some employers are taking a hard line. United Airlines told employees last week that those who obtain religious exemptions will be put on unpaid leave until new coronavirus testing procedures are in place.

In Los Angeles, Police Chief Michel Moore said he is waiting for guidance from the city personnel department regarding the exemptions. The city has mandated that municipal employees get vaccinated by Oct. 5 unless they are granted a medical or religious exemption. A group of LAPD employees is suing over the policy.

"Let me be absolutely clear: We will not tolerate the abuse of these exemptions by those who simply don't want to get vaccinated," Los Angeles Mayor Eric Garcetti said. "To anyone thinking about filing a disingenuous exemption request, I strongly urge you to reconsider."

In Washington State, approximately 60,000 State employees are subject to a mandate issued by Gov. Jay Inslee that they be fully vaccinated by Oct. 18 or lose their job, unless they obtain a medical or religious exemption and receive an accommodation that allows them to remain employees.

As of Tuesday, more than 3,800 workers had requested religious exemptions. So far, 737 have been approved, but officials stressed that an exemption does not guarantee continued employment.

Once the exemption is approved, each agency has to evaluate whether the employee can still do the job with an accommodation while ensuring a safe workplace. Seven accommodations so far have been granted.

Inslee spokeswoman Tara Lee said the process "may help distinguish between a sincerely held personal belief and a sincerely held religious belief."

Conway Regional Health System

In Arkansas, about 5 per cent of the staff at the privately run Conway Regional Health System has requested religious or medical exemptions.

The hospital responded by sending employees a form that lists a multitude of common medicines—including Tylenol, Pepto-Bismol, Preparation H and Tums—that it said were developed or tested using fetal cell lines.

The form asks people to sign it and attest that "my sincerely held religious belief is consistent and true and I do not use or will not use" any of the listed medications.

In a statement, Conway Regional Health President and CEO Matt Troup said: "Staff who are sincere ... should have no hesitancy with agreeing to the list of medicines listed."

Periodical and Internet Sources Bibliography

The following articles have been selected to supplement the diverse views presented in this chapter.

Joss Fong, "How American Conservatives Turned Against the Vaccine," VOX, February 23, 2022. https://www.vox.com/22947498/partisan-pandemic-polarization-coronavirus-vaccine.

William A. Galston, "For Covid-19 Vaccinations, Party Affiliation Matters More Than Race and Ethnicity," Brookings, October 1, 2021. https://www.brookings.edu/blog/fixgov/2021/10/01/for-covid-19-vaccinations-party-affiliation-matters-more-than-race-and-ethnicity/.

Jon Greenberg, "Few religions ban vaccination, but that counts little for religious exemptions," Politifact, October 6, 2021. https://www.politifact.com/factchecks/2021/oct/06/anthony-fauci/few-religions-ban-vaccination-counts-little-religi/

Olga Khazan, "The Tucker Carlson Fans That Got Vaxxed," *Atlantic*, August 9, 2021. https://www.theatlantic.com/politics/archive/2021/08/why-so-many-republicans-wont-get-vaccinated/619659/.

Colleen Long and Andrew DeMillo, "As Covid-19 Vaccination Mandates Rise, Religious Exemptions Grow," Associated Press, September 15, 2021. https://apnews.com/article/joe-biden-health-religion-los-angeles-arkansas-3ba53f2f00e1ab7105d7d128f2b1e65d.

Lee McIntyre, "Why Are So Many Republicans Refusing Vaccination? Because Russia is Telling Them To," *Baltimore Sun*, July 30, 2021. https://www.baltimoresun.com/opinion/op-ed/bs-ed-op-0801-covid-disinformation-russia-20210730-5tz4sglw6jadrajptaeismgifm-story.html.

Philip Pullella, "Pope Urges Covid Inoculations, Says Vaccines are Humanity's Friends," Reuters, September 15, 2021. https://www.reuters.com/business/healthcare-pharmaceuticals/pope-urges-covid-inoculations-says-vaccines-are-humanitys-friends-2021-09-15/.

OPPOSING VIEWPOINTS® SERIES

Chapter 4

What Is the Future for Vaccines?

Chapter Preface

Medical treatments have advanced steadily since the early days of vaccines. An understanding of what causes disease and how to combat it will continue to increase, while treatments will continue to be refined and improved.

Viable questions emerge. What should be done to enhance the field of vaccine science? How can misinformation and conspiracy theories be thwarted? Can humans learn to avoid zoonotic disease? Will countries around the world learn to fully cooperate against future pandemics? As the global response to the COVID-19 virus demonstrates, a concerted effort must be organized now to be prepared for pandemics and the associated vaccines of the future.

Almost certainly, there will always be a fraction of any population who are outspoken agents against science, medicine, and governments. This anti-science, anti-vaccine, anti-government attitude must be rectified when public health is at risk.

Viewpoint authors in this chapter address the ability of medicine and science to communicate to laypeople the importance of vaccines to keep individuals safe from disease and disability. Some point to the necessity of social media to change practices that enable misinformation to proliferate and cause confusion and mistrust. Others argue that medical workers, governments, and trusted community individuals must actively seek to correct erroneous thinking and feeling that contributes to conspiracy theories and misguided beliefs, which in turn cause people to turn away from safe, viable, medical treatments.

Viewpoint 1

> *"There is only 'one health,' the health of all living organisms in a global ecosystem that, when rapidly altered and imbalanced, puts us all at risk for future pandemics."*

"One Health" Is a Global Plan to Prevent Future Pandemics

Hélène Carabin

In the following viewpoint Hélène Carabin analyzes the health management plan, "One Health." Carabine outlines the aims of this proposed global health system, detailing how it would integrate existing systems and how it would enhance existing programs. Hélène Carabin is a professor of epidemiology at the University of Montreal in Canada.

As you read, consider the following questions:

1. According to the author, what amount of emerging human infectious diseases is based in animal origins?
2. What three global agencies collaborate in the "One Health" program?
3. What has the World Health Assembly proposed?

"One Health: A Crucial Approach to Preventing and Preparing for Future Pandemics," by Hélène Carabin, The Conversation, December 23, 2021. https://theconversation.com/one-health-a-crucial-approach-to-preventing-and-preparing-for-future-pandemics-173637. Licensed under CC BY-ND 4.0 International.

One Health is a concept that emerged in the early 2000s that recognizes the interconnections and health interdependencies among humans, other animals and the shared environments in which we live and interact.

In some cases, these shared environments make it possible for infectious agents—such as viruses—to adapt and move between species. Zoonotic diseases are infectious diseases that are transmitted to humans from animals or vice versa. They include COVID-19, Ebola and HIV, as well as much older diseases like tuberculosis.

Significant changes in our global ecosystem, such as loss of natural habitats, are altering the way humans interact with other animals and the environment, leading to the emergence of new zoonotic diseases. It is currently estimated that approximately three-quarters of emerging infectious diseases in humans have an animal origin.

The COVID-19 pandemic underscores that human health is fundamentally interconnected with the health of other animals (domestic and wild) throughout our shared environment. There is only "one health," the health of all living organisms in a global ecosystem that, when rapidly altered and imbalanced, puts us all at risk for future pandemics.

Global Collaboration

There is growing recognition that gaps in local, national and global governance contribute to the emergence and re-emergence of zoonotic diseases. A broad collaboration has been underway to address this for several years.

The tripartite One Health collaboration between the Food and Agriculture Organization of the United Nations (FAO), the World Organisation for Animal Health (OIE) and the World Health Organization (WHO) has, since 2010, been one of the most significant high-level initiatives to strengthen the adoption of the One Health approach to human-animal-environmental health.

First developed to address the threat of antimicrobial resistance, the tripartite also published a guide for the control of zoonotic diseases before the emergence of the COVID-19 pandemic.

The United Nations Environment Programme collaborated with the FAO-OIE-WHO tripartite to establish the One Health High Level Expert Panel (OHHLEP) on Dec. 1. OHHLEP defines the One Health approach as:

> One Health is an integrated, unifying approach that aims to achieve optimal and sustainable health outcomes for people, animals, and ecosystems. It recognizes that the health of humans, domestic and wild animals, plants, and the wider environment (our ecosystems) are closely linked and inter-dependent.
>
> The approach mobilizes multiple sectors, disciplines and communities at all levels of society to work together to tackle threats to health and ecosystems, while addressing our collective needs for healthy food, water, energy and air, taking action on climate change, and promoting sustainable development.

An Essential Part of the Pandemic Treaty

The World Health Assembly—the decision-making body of the WHO—proposed establishing a pandemic treaty at a special session held from Nov. 29 to Dec. 1.

Under international law, a treaty is a legally binding instrument. An international treaty on pandemics would mandate and support WHO member states to build national, regional and global pandemic capacity and resilience through improved prevention, prediction, preparedness and response.

I am a university professor and the Tier 1 Canada Research Chair in Epidemiology and One Health. As the co-senior author, I am writing on behalf of the authors of a guidance note submitted with the Pandemic Treaty proposal. In it, we explain the central role that an equity-oriented One Health approach could play in pandemic prevention and preparedness.

Addressing risk factors at the human-animal-environment interface—like encroachment of natural habitats by humans—is key to prevention. Enabling better preparedness by, for example, establishing and maintaining highly integrated multi-species surveillance systems, will also require co-ordinating the actions of countries while integrating the medical, public health, veterinary, agronomy, engineering, computer sciences, social sciences and environmental sectors and many more.

There is little integration of One Health principles in existing international treaties and regulations. In our guidance note, we recommend their integration into a future treaty on pandemics. We also explain how this would complement and strengthen the connectivity (the ability to link, communicate and co-ordinate) between existing international agreements.

We propose developing universal metrics for evaluating how the One Health approach is being implemented in different countries.

We recommend fully integrating the One Health approach into all key elements of a pandemic treaty—prevention, surveillance, preparedness and response—and including commitments to financial support. This integration must be done with equity and solidarity in mind to ensure that all will benefit from pandemic prevention. Access to human, animal and ecosystem health diagnostics, treatments and services must be guaranteed and universal.

The inclusion of One Health in a pandemic treaty will help ensure collaboration between and across disciplines and sectors. It will require a strong commitment to increase our One Health knowledge through research and translating its results for a wider audience, with support from the international community.

Our policy brief also recommends the creation of a permanent global structure to ensure funding and implementation, similar to existing structures for biodiversity and climate change.

A pandemic treaty that incorporates One Health would advance pandemic prevention and preparedness, as well as human, animal and environmental health. It would contribute to the protection of biodiversity, reduce activities that increase the risk of pandemics such as illicit wildlife trafficking and harmful land-use changes, and would also avoid catastrophic global financial losses. Such a treaty would also improve the lives of all living beings by reducing the burden on animal and human health care as well as pressure on ecosystems and agricultural lands, and on small producers and communities.

In his closing address to the special assembly, WHO Director-General Tedros Adhanom Ghebreyesus said: "We are one humanity. We have one planet. We have one health."

What About Canada?

A treaty that integrates the One Health approach to prevention and preparedness for future pandemics at all levels of government, in research, and in the organization of interventions is a major step forward on a global scale.

Canada recently established an interdisciplinary action research network called Global 1HN. It aims to strengthen Canadian leadership in improving the global governance of infectious diseases and antimicrobial resistance. In doing so, it supports the importance of incorporating a One Health approach within a pandemic treaty.

Negotiations underway for such a treaty mark a critical step forward in protecting not only the health of Canadians, but also the interdependent health of all living beings.

Viewpoint 2

> *"The central dogma of the anti-vaccine ideology is that vaccines cause autism and other bad health effects, and that governments and the pharmaceutical industry knowingly suppress this information."*

Vaccines: Separating Sense from Nonsense

Jonathan Jarry

In the following viewpoint Jonathan Jarry analyzes the changes occurring in the anti-vaxx movement. Jarry maintains that from a "vaccines cause autism" standpoint to "big pharma is bad and natural immunity is better," the anti-vaccine movement is using social media to cloud true science. He further argues that scientific facts are being lost to a robust social media campaign infiltrating large numbers of online followers and convincing the vaccine hesitant to become more confused and unsure of scientific fact. Jonathan Jarry is a science communicator with the McGill University Office for Science and Society.

As you read, consider the following questions:

1. According to the author, which groups are joining anti-vaccine protestors?
2. What is natural immunity theory?
3. According to the viewpoint, what distinction belongs to former President Donald Trump?

"The Anti-Vaccine Movement in 2020," by Jonathan Jarry, McGill University's Office for Science and Society, May 22, 2020. Reprinted by permission.

What does an antivaxxer and a far-right activist have in common? If the thought of someone who opposes vaccines brings to mind tie-dye shirts and tree hugging, your answer may be "nothing." But clearly, some do have a commonality: protesting the COVID-19 lockdowns. Coverage from these protests often show people holding signs slapped with antivaccine rhetoric next to pro-militia activists and white supremacists. This phenomenon can also be seen among homeschoolers according to Anne Borden, a pro-vaccine homeschooler who fights against phony autism cures. "The first antivaxxers I ever met were left-leaning unschoolers when I was an unschooled teenager. They were very much a part of the early efforts to 'stop the Food and Drug Administration' from regulating alternative medicine. What has happened in recent years is that this demographic of homeschooling is being now recruited by the radical right on social media, and some are turning right. And this is very concerning."

This may leave you wondering just what is happening to the anti-vaccine movement in 2020.

The central dogma of the anti-vaccine ideology is that vaccines cause autism and other bad health effects, and that governments and the pharmaceutical industry knowingly suppress this information. This tenet, we easily imagine, is tightly wedded to the political left. It's a hippy-dippy attitude, we often think, borne out of an irrational fear of chemicals, and there are indeed prominent spokespeople for the movement who fit this sketch. Joe Mercola made his fortune selling natural health products and has contributed more than $2.9 million to the National Vaccine Information Center in the U.S., an anti-vaccine advocacy group. There is Robert F. Kennedy, Jr., a Democrat and environmentalist, who is a major public figure on the anti-vaccination scene as the chairman of the Children's Health Defense. This branch of the movement shows a distrust of pharmaceutical companies and a pursuit of purity. Their wrongful idea that nature is inherently good ends up framing their thinking, which is why in the age of COVID we read about their "natural immunity theory": that barriers to germs, like physical distancing and masks, weaken our immune system. Vaccines are just one more synthetic loaded gun aimed at our immune system, they say. The embedding of antivaxx sentiment within this nature worship is familiar to many of us. But there is a segment of the anti-vaccination movement on the far right, drawn to its libertarian streak of distrusting the government, and there exists at least one prominent bridge between leftist antivaxxers and the political right in the United States: Donald Trump.

Before associating with the Republicans and as far back as 2007, Trump had publicly expressed the erroneous belief that vaccines cause autism. He has helped raise money over the years for his friend Bob Wright, who founded the charity Autism Speaks whose stance on vaccines has been deemed "controversial." And Trump himself invited Robert F. Kennedy, Jr., to chair a commission on vaccine safety (which ended up dying on the vine). Trump, it should be pointed out, is the first American president to be on the record as having anti-vaccine views, an influence that cannot be ignored. A survey involving Americans who voted in the 2016 presidential election revealed that Trump voters expressed more vaccine concern (specifically about the MMR vaccine, wrongly linked to autism) than non-Trump voters, a result which the authors conclude was explained by their conspiracist ideation. This association between the current right-wing of American politics and questioning the value and safety of vaccines can also be seen in Gallup polls. For the years 2001, 2015 and 2019, the percentage of Democrats who say it is either extremely or very important for parents to vaccinate their children has moved from 97% to 88% to 92%. For the same time points, Republicans went from 93% to 82% to 79%.

Beyond political affiliation, researchers can shed some additional light on who an antivaxxer tends to be and how they think. Interviews with Australian parents who reject vaccines revealed they see themselves as virtuous but oppressed, and vaccinators are perceived as an "Unhealthy Other." Those who

WHO Says No to Mandatory Vaccinations

The World Health Organization (WHO) warns against mandatory vaccinations unless all other options have been exhausted.

Dr Hans Kluge, the Europe Director of WHO told a press conference today that vaccinations should not be made mandatory "if you haven't reached out first to the communities."

"Mandates around vaccination are an absolute last resort and only applicable when all other feasible options to improve vaccination uptake have been exhausted."

Kluge admitted that such measures had been proven effective in some environments, to increase vaccine uptake.

However, the effect that mandating vaccination could have on public confidence and public trust, as well as vaccination uptake, must be considered.

While cases and deaths have more than doubled in the past two months, COVID-19 deaths have remained significantly below previous peaks. Kluge says that the mortality would have been far worse without vaccination. 55% of all people in Europe and Central Asia are fully vaccinated and 43 out of 53 countries now offer an additional booster dose to their most vulnerable populations.

Dr Kluge pointed out new research conducted by WHO Europe and the European Centre for Disease Prevention and Control, which found that from December 2020 to November 2021, at least 470,000 lives were directly saved through COVID-19 vaccination.

"This is an overwhelming affirmation of the value of vaccines and science, a testimony to government and healthcare worker commitment and most of all a great recognition of the public's acceptance and support to tackling this pandemic," Dr Kluge said.

He said that Europeans needed to shift from "reaction" to "stabilization" mode in this crisis. Five pandemic stabilizers were needed to keep mortality down, including increasing vaccine uptake, administering a booster, doubling the rate of mask-wearing indoor and ventilating crowded spaces.

"WHO: Mandatory Vaccinations Are a Last Resort," The United Nations, July 12, 2021.

reject vaccines may have a skewed perception of the risks posed by them and the diseases they prevent, with some evidence showing that Internet searches may increase the perception that childhood vaccines are risky. And a large investigation into the anti-vaccination phenomenon, conducted in 24 countries by a team at the University of Queensland, revealed a strong pattern: people who reported more conspiratorial beliefs tended to be more anti-vaccine. This association was particularly strong in Western nations, like Canada and the U.S. Next in line was the link between anti-vaccination attitudes and the resistance to having their freedom taken away from them. The authors report that "more conservative participants also had stronger antivaccination attitudes." What was not linked to antivaxx beliefs was education.

The prototypical antivaxxer described above, though, does not exist in a vacuum. The people who espouse these views can find each other quite easily because of the existence of an important conduit that allows their claims, anxieties and incitements to spread: social media. Even though social media giants have said they would crack down on vaccine misinformation, anti-vaccine communities quickly adapt to the new rules, like a guided virus mutating with a purpose. For example, the word "vaccine" disappears in the name of their group, replaced by "medical freedom." And according to a recent massive analysis of 100 million Facebook users worldwide, online supporters of anti-vaccine views have been more successful by some measures than those of us publicly supporting vaccines. They are smaller numerically but occupy a more central position in the network; they are heavily involved with clusters of Facebook users who haven't made up their mind about vaccines; and they offer a wide variety of "potentially attractive" stories (about safety concerns, about government conspiracies, about natural immunity) that can attract a greater diversity of people compared to pro-vaccine messaging which tends to be one-note. This diversity is also encouraged by social media companies.

Platforms like Facebook and YouTube want to hold onto your eyeballs so they recommend other content. Renee DiResta, a security researcher, told BuzzFeed News that as she joined more anti-vaccine parenting groups on Facebook for the purpose of investigating them, the platform recommended more and more conspiracist groups: about chemtrails, about the flat Earth, about the Pizzagate conspiracy theory. She called this phenomenon "radicalization via the recommendation engine." And as Anne Borden was telling me, there is active cross-pollination happening on social media with the far right. "Right-wing movements have deeply infiltrated the social media spaces of the antivaxx and vaccine-hesitant homeschoolers and alt-schoolers. They recruit in antivaxx and Facebook groups related to complementary and alternative medicine."

What These Concerns and Conspiracy Theories May Mean for the Future

When we pull at this big ball of conspiracy theories and pro-freedom sentiment, we can find some genuine concerns buried inside. Jon Perry, the founder of the Stated Clearly science communication project, pointed me in the direction of a Facebook meme declaring that its poster would not be "vaccinated (chipped) for the coronavirus." "The meme," he told me, "is a mixed bag of legitimate concerns about tracking devices, a justifiable mistrust of billionaires and large organizations, common knowledge that most large nations dabble (or have dabbled) in bio-weapons research, a far less warranted (but not totally baseless) fear of new vaccines, and many more, all combined with a horrible confusion about medical patents and virus naming structures." A project like ID2020, aimed at providing everyone with a secure digital identification, can be twisted by a distrustful, pattern-seeking mind into a cover for Bill Gates' nefarious plan to monitor every human being. The fact that multiple coronavirus vaccines use the virus' RNA can be misinterpreted into the fear that vaccines will mutate our own DNA. Justified worries are fed by misunderstandings and further amplified by a conspiracist mindset in online communities cross-pollinated by radical political actors, leading to progressive vaccine-hesitant parents holding hands with the anti-lockdown movement. Like a big ball of colourful rubber bands, these disparate-looking actors share an underlying property and end up sticking together.

While this big wobbly ball looks overwhelming, there are discreet actions pro-vaccine people and organizations can take to minimize the damage caused by anti-vaccine attitudes, and because these attitudes tend to be tied to the belief in a grand conspiracy, the recent publication of the Conspiracy Theory Handbook can be of help. When addressing members of the public unlikely to endorse conspiracy theories, the Handbook recommends empowering people with facts, uncovering the bad logic in the initial argument, linking to fact-checking websites, and exposing the lack of credibility of the sources of these theories. Trying to reach extremists, on the other hand, is usually a fool's errand; personally, I'd rather address the people on the fence and we have preliminary evidence that empathy and really listening to the concerns of vaccine-hesitant parents can improve their attitudes toward vaccines.

If safe and effective vaccines against the new coronavirus end up being approved (which is not a guarantee, though over 90 experimental vaccines are at various testing stages), I wonder how much public confidence will have been eroded by this reenergized anti-vaccine movement and their radical allies. In the past decade, the United States has seen a 10% overall decline in the number of parents who feel it's extremely or very important to vaccinate their children (from 94% in 2001 to 84% in 2019), with 11% saying they think vaccines are more dangerous than the disease they are meant to prevent. Meanwhile, in 2015, almost two in five respondents to a Canadian survey agreed that the science on vaccinations isn't quite clear. What these numbers capture is not just antivaxxers, however. Their movement is a small and vocal minority, but its fear-based messaging reaches a larger segment of the population: the vaccine hesitant. And people on the fence about vaccines are now being served an incredible buffet of prickly anxieties: from genuine concerns that a coronavirus vaccine may be rushed to the loud cries of “my body, my temple”, all the way to stories of Bill Gates’ evil plan to depopulate the world, with the occasional viral video like Plandemic fuelling this unease with a veneer of respectability. How much damage this ever-growing ball will cause on its way down the slope is anyone’s guess, but we have genuine reason to be worried.

Viewpoint 3

"The exhaustive amount of scientific evidence confirming that vaccines are safe should ease anyone's concerns about how they're made and tested."

Vaccines Are Safe and Effective

New York State Department of Health

In the following viewpoint the New York State Department of Health (DoH) provides an overview of vaccine development and safety. The author breaks down the development process and outlines the continued testing and watchfulness that occurs after a vaccine is out for general use by the public. The author also touches on the chemical thimerosal, which was once accused of causing problems in vaccinated children but is no longer a component of pediatric vaccinations. The New York State Department of Health is a governmental agency of the state of New York.

As you read, consider the following questions:

1. Which U.S. agency is charged with the safety of vaccines as reported in the viewpoint?
2. What is in a vaccine that causes people's bodies to produce an immune response?
3. As stated in the viewpoint, which vaccine is made quickly each year?

"The Science Behind Vaccine Research and Testing," New York State Department of Health. Reprinted by permission.

The creation of a vaccine involves scientists and medical experts from around the world, and it usually requires 10 to 15 years of research before the vaccine is made available to the general public. The first step of this extensive process involves several years of laboratory research, in which scientists and researchers identify an antigen that can prevent a disease.

Once the test vaccine has been cleared for further investigation by the U.S. Food and Drug Administration, at least three more phases of thorough clinical trials are conducted on human volunteers to test vaccine efficacy, to determine appropriate dosage, and to monitor for adverse side effects, etc. These trials usually take several more years to complete. The last phase involves a test group of up to tens of thousands of human volunteers. Unsure if this is a large enough test group? Consider this—medicines in the United States also go through incredible scrutiny, but their test subject sample sizes are three times smaller than vaccine test subject groups.

But that's not the end of it: Once approved, the FDA continues to closely monitor the vaccine . It tests everything from batches of the vaccine to the production process and the facilities for safety. The FDA also conducts ongoing monitoring of vaccine reactions. Numerous agencies also work together on a global level to track, collect and analyze data, to make sure these vaccines are, and remain, safe for the general population. For more information on vaccine coordination and monitoring, visit the CDC's page on Why It's Important to Monitor Vaccine Safety and the Immunization Safety Office.

Unlike other vaccines, which typically take 10 to 15 years of research, development and testing before being approved by the U.S. Food and Drug Administration (FDA), seasonal flu vaccines are developed on an annual basis. While the antigen changes in the flu vaccine every year, the manufacturing process remains the same and is founded on ongoing virus tracking around the world. Scientists can determine which flu virus is most likely to circulate during the next flu season, and once identified, can change the antigen but keep everything else in the vaccine the same. This process builds on time-proven techniques and allows the medical community to respond quickly to protect the public from changing flu viruses. For more information visit The Facts Behind Vaccine Safety

The exhaustive amount of scientific evidence confirming that vaccines are safe should ease anyone's concerns about how they're made and tested. The flu vaccine is no exception.

Vaccines build your body's immune system so that, in the future, it's able to fight against a specific disease. Today's arsenal of vaccines protect us against many types of diseases that we could still encounter in our lives. Many of these diseases can be crippling or even deadly if you come into contact with them and aren't vaccinated.

Vaccine Ingredients

Injecting something into your body can be concerning for some, especially when you're unsure of what's inside the needle. We're here to take the mystery out of a vaccine's ingredients.

A vaccine contains a part of a germ (bacteria or virus) that is called an antigen. The antigen has already been killed or disabled before it's used to make the vaccine, so it can't make you sick. Antigens are substances, often a protein, that stimulate the body to produce an immune response to protect itself against attacks from future actual disease exposure. In addition, vaccines contain other ingredients that make them safer and more effective, including preservatives, adjuvants, additives and residuals of the vaccine production process. Because specific ingredients are necessary to make a vaccine, even though they are eventually removed, trace amounts can still remain. These residuals can include small amounts of antibiotics and egg or yeast protein. The American Academy of Pediatrics also provides a good explanation about what's inside the vaccine needle.

If you're a parent concerned that your child may be exposed to too many antigens, there's no need to worry: Today's vaccines contain far less antigens than in the past, thanks to advances in biomedical science. Additionally, children's bodies are well equipped to handle many antigens at the same time. A healthy baby can accommodate multiple vaccinations because vaccines, and the antigens they contain are designed for babies' immune systems. In fact, babies can handle significantly more antigens than those that are found in vaccines.

A few years ago, much attention was placed on thimerosal, an organic form of mercury (also called ethylmercury) that prevents vaccines from being contaminated. This form of mercury is different from methylmercury, which can damage the nervous system. Although thimerosal has been shown to be safe, now all routine childhood vaccines are produced in thimerosal-free form. This includes the flu vaccine.

Viewpoint 4

> *"The post was flagged as part of Facebook's efforts to combat false news and misinformation on its News Feed."*

For the Future, False Claims on Social Media About Vaccines Must Be Stopped

Samantha Putterman

In the following viewpoint Samantha Putterman analyzes a claim made via video clip on social media by a virologist that the COVID-19 vaccination causes variants of the virus to occur. Putterman systematically debunks the false accusation. By using testimony from several scientists and health experts, Putterman systematically fact checks the claim and handily tosses it into the garbage can of false claims. Samantha Putterman is a fact-checker with PolitiFact and based in New York.

As you read, consider the following questions:

1. Who is making the claim about COVID-19 causing variants according to Putterman?
2. Does the misleading video appear to be doctored?
3. What is one reason that supports the case for this video being false as stated in this viewpoint?

"COVID-19 Vaccines Are Creating the Coronavirus Variants," by Samantha Putterman, Politifact, May 28, 2021. Reprinted by permission.

This is a new one.

Instead of the established understanding that vaccines help reduce the spread of COVID-19, and thereby decrease the likelihood that the virus will be able to mutate enough to create new variants, a new claim circulating online posits that it's the vaccines that are creating the variants.

The claim comes from French virologist Luc Montagnier, a joint recipient of the Nobel Prize in 2008 for discovering HIV. But Montagnier has been in the news since for sharing what some scientists characterize as pseudoscientific statements, most recently relating to misinformation about the coronavirus.

Montagnier makes the claim in a 2-minute video spreading on Facebook that's spoken in French with English subtitles. It bears the watermark of the RAIR Foundation, which describes itself as a "grassroots activist organization" that's working to "combat the threats from Islamic supremacists, radical leftists and their allies."

In the video, Montagnier calls the vaccination program for COVID-19 "an unacceptable mistake" because, according to him, "it is the vaccination that is creating the variants."

He adds: "For the China virus there are antibodies created by the vaccine. What does the virus do? Does it die or find another solution? The new variants are a production and result from the vaccination."

The post was flagged as part of Facebook's efforts to combat false news and misinformation on its News Feed.

First, it's important to note that we found no evidence that this video is doctored.

Bethan John, a French speaker and social media journalist for the misinformation research organization First Draft, wrote up an analysis of the video and says the clip of Montagnier was posted on alternative video sharing platform Odysee by HOLD-UP Média, a group behind a viral French documentary-style video about the pandemic that's been debunked by fact-checkers.

John reported that the video's misleading narrative that the vaccines create variants has been gaining traction in France for several weeks. Other First Draft researchers also found the video circulating in Spanish and Portugese and said the subtitles matched the claims Montagnier is seen making in the video, though there are a lot of sharp editing cuts throughout.

But while the video appears legitimate, what Montagnier said in it is not.

First, several of the variants that are circulating in the global population emerged before COVID-19 vaccines were widely available, like B.1.1.7, the variant that emerged in the United Kingdom in September 2020. Second, the vaccines help reduce the spread of the virus, therefore decreasing the likelihood that it will mutate and create new variants.

The video's claim is a distortion of the factual premise that slow vaccine uptake in a population can lead to the development of variants.

Viruses try to create variants in order to escape immunity—but that's any immunity—vaccine-induced or natural, which arises from being infected.

The difference is that people who are vaccinated are better protected against such variants.

"The virus is always going to try to evolve to promote its own survival," said Dr. Sarah Fortune, chair of the Immunology and Infectious Diseases department at Harvard T.H. Chan School of Public Health. "It doesn't mean people shouldn't get vaccinated. The virus is going to try to evolve to escape natural immunity, even if you choose not to get vaccinated."

She added: "Either people are going to get sick and get COVID-19, and the virus tries to escape that immune selection, or people can be vaccinated and the virus is going to try to escape that immune selection. Avoiding vaccination is not going to limit the evolution of the virus."

Antibody-Dependent Enhancement

In the video, Montagnier also discusses a phenomenon called "antibody-dependent enhancement" as a concern with the COVID-19 vaccines. That's a phenomenon that happens when antibodies produced by an infection or a vaccine bind to the viral pathogen, but don't kill it. Sometimes called "ADE," it can cause people with antibodies to have more severe symptoms should they end up getting infected later.

But the video fails to mention that this has not been observed with COVID-19 or any of the vaccines that have been developed to prevent it.

ADE was initially a concern contemplated by scientists when they were creating COVID-19 vaccines. Animal studies were designed to specifically look for signs of ADE, and did not find any evidence of it. There has also been no sign of it happening in the real world rollout of the vaccines.

"With lots and lots of experience with use of antibodies therapeutically, we've seen no evidence of enhancement," Dr. Stuart Ray, a professor at Johns Hopkins University's medical school, told the Associated Press in a related fact-check. "We also worried about the possibility that people who were reinfected might have more severe infection, akin to the situation we've seen with dengue virus, and that also hasn't been borne out. So there's really no basis for the claim that's being ascribed to Dr. Montagnier."

Montagnier's Pseudoscience Claims

Shortly after winning the Nobel Prize, Montagnier started to make headlines when he claimed that a "good immune system" was enough to protect people against AIDS. He has also become known for being anti-vaccination and pro-homeopathy and believes that "water has memory," a theory that has been discredited by the scientific community.

In 2017, in response to Montagnier's claims that vaccines are poisonous, over 100 academic scientists wrote an open letter that said, "We, academics of medicine, cannot accept that one of our peers is using his Nobel Prize [status] to spread dangerous health messages outside of his field of knowledge," according to the French news website Connexion.

Our Ruling

A video on Facebook shows French virologist Luc Montagnier claiming that the COVID-19 vaccines create the variants.

The COVID-19 vaccines help reduce the spread of the virus, decreasing the likelihood that it will mutate and create new variants. Several coronavirus variants emerged before the vaccines were rolled out in late 2020.

Slow vaccine uptake can cause more variants, since the virus continually looks to evolve and escape any immunity—natural or vaccine-induced. Public health experts say this doesn't mean that people shouldn't get vaccinated, but just the opposite, as faster uptake slows this from happening and will leave people better protected from the virus in the process.

We rate this False.

Viewpoint 5

> *"Can the government go against private interests to protect the public interest?"*

Pharmaceutical Patents Stand in the Way of Making Important Vaccines Accessible Around the World

Sophia Crabbe Field

In the following viewpoint Sophia Crabbe Field reports on attempts to pressure pharmaceutical companies to make vaccines accessible globally in an effort to end the COVID-19 pandemic by temporarily waiving patents on vaccines. Not surprisingly, big pharma is resistant to such waivers, as are many governments that have traditionally protected and supported pharmaceutical companies. Sophia Crabbe Field is the associate editor of Democracy: A Journal of Ideas.

As you read, consider the following questions:

1. What is the TRIPS waiver?
2. Why is global vaccine equity important?
3. Why is the waiver alone not enough to deliver vaccines around the world?

"Global Health Activists Say It's Time for Big Pharma to Make a Sacrifice," by Sophia Crabbe Field, Waging Nonviolence, July 29, 2021. https://wagingnonviolence.org/2021/07/europe-blocks-access-covid-vaccines-renew-pressure-biden/. Licensed under CC BY-4.0 International.

On July 15, Andrew Goldstein, a primary care doctor in New York City, stepped out for his lunch break, dressed in his scrubs, to take part in a march headed toward the German Permanent Mission to the United Nations, accompanied by around 200 other protesters. That week, protests were held nationwide to mark Angela Merkel's final visit to the United States and to bring attention to her key role in blocking the TRIPS waiver for the COVID-19 vaccine at the World Trade Organization.

As a doctor, Goldstein explained, "I feel that I'm complicit, and I don't want to be, in a system that's very profit-driven. So I think it's important for health workers to show up." In front of Pfizer's New York headquarters, protesters later blocked traffic in an act of civil disobedience. At the same time, a die-in took place in front of the White House in Washington, D.C. There, activists laid out body bags in front of a giant puppet of Angela Merkel. Protests were also held in front of more than a dozen consular offices across the country

The European Union, and Germany more specifically, is seen as the main stumbling block in the fight for the TRIPS waiver, which was first proposed by the governments of South Africa and India in October 2020 and has now become a rallying cry for global vaccine equity. The waiver would temporarily remove certain rules under the WTO's Trade-Related Aspects of Intellectual Property Rights Agreement, or TRIPS, to allow for the lifting of patents on vaccines, equipment and technologies related to COVID-19.

On May 5, in a widely heralded victory for the access to medicines movement, the Biden administration announced that it would support a waiver on vaccines. Even though what President Biden proposed was much more limited than the proposal put forth by South Africa and India, the waiver had become "respectable." "Suddenly it was mainstream," said Jaume Vidal, senior policy advisor at Health Action International. This move was also seen as an unprecedented shift for a country that has long supported the most stringent possible protections for the pharmaceutical industry.

Arthur Stamoulis, executive director of Citizens Trade Campaign, who helped organize the die-in as well as other events during Merkel's visit, noted that campaigners on both sides of the Atlantic saw Merkel's valedictory final tour to the United States as "a prime opportunity to put direct pressure on her and to encourage the administration to do the same." Activists were pleased with the attention garnered in the press. Stamoulis pointed to the fact that the New York Times' lead story on Merkel's visit featured a photo of the protest in Washington, D.C. and images of the protests featured heavily in German media.

Despite these victories, however, there was disappointment in the lack of a direct political outcome. The Merkel-Biden press conference at the end of the visit made no mention of the TRIPS waiver. According to Stamoulis, the issue reportedly came up in private with Biden, "but there was clearly no resolution to it." With elections in Germany set for September, activists see little chance of Merkel changing positions; there was a lot of pride in Germany around the success of the BioNTech vaccine and there is a strong ideological belief in her party in the importance of patents for innovation.

But with Merkel's exit imminent, some are looking elsewhere on Germany's political stage, including toward the German Green Party, which is currently climbing in the polls and could form part of a governing majority come September. Lara Dovifat, international campaign manager for Doctors Without Borders' Access to Medicines Campaign, who is based in Germany, sees the success of the Green Party as a "prime opportunity to make the issue of waiving patents and creating better access to life-saving medical tools" an election issue.

As activists in the United States take stock of recent events, they may look to pivot toward renewed pressure on the Biden administration. Since his May 5 announcement, many feel that the president is not doing enough. Biden invited the CEO of Pfizer as his guest to the G7 in June, and the United States has reportedly remained silent on the issue at recent WTO TRIPS Council meetings.

However, Arthur Stamoulis believes that with the Delta variant advancing quickly, the potential threat of more lockdowns, and California even reinstituting its mask mandate, Americans might be forced to finally reckon with the fact that "no one is safe until everyone is safe." Brook Baker, a senior policy analyst at Health Gap, would like to see Biden work directly with the initial sponsors of the waiver, South Africa and India, to force Europe to negotiate.

The Waiver in Europe

Marc Botenga is a Belgian member of the European Parliament where he is part of The Left coalition. In March 2020, he brought a resolution before Parliament in support of the TRIPS waiver. Having spent time in South Africa while working in global health, he was inspired by members of the Treatment Action Campaign, who successfully advocated for access to HIV/AIDS medications in the late 1990s and early 2000s. He saw how "patents and intellectual property rights in general were a massive break on access to the treatments that we had at the time." This time, he said, "Either you would have strong public action on intellectual property rights or the dynamics were going to be very similar."

When Botenga initiated his proposal, he continued, "There seemed to be this window of opportunity because you had a number of important policy figures in the European Union actually declaring that the vaccine should be a common good." His resolution supporting the waiver passed with a strong majority in the European Parliament in June.

Yet when he first brought forward the resolution, Botenga said he felt "very lonely," and thought that there was "no way we're going to win this inside Parliament." He credits the work of grassroots activists in the eventual success of the proposal, noting the role of the People's Vaccine Alliance in Europe, which has organized rallies around the continent and has used social media to mobilize citizen engagement, as well as Doctors Without Borders, in influencing many of his colleagues.

Meanwhile, Jaume Vidal emphasized the positive response of parliamentarians with whom he began meeting with in November 2020. "When you do advocacy, it's rare when you can say 'we won,' but in this case we won," Vidal added. "We approved the resolution that pharma didn't want approved."

Unfortunately, this victory remains mostly a symbolic one, as parliament doesn't set policy at the WTO. That is the job of European Commission, which represents the interests of the European Union on the global stage and has been setting the agenda with regards to Europe's position on the waiver. Doctors Without Borders' requests for meetings with commissioners have been repeatedly denied, though they have spoken with lower level officials. Dimitri Eynikel, coordinator of the policy team for the Access to Medicines Campaign in Europe, said this is frustrating, particularly when Doctors Without Borders was so directly involved in helping to deliver aid to EU countries during the pandemic.

They also know that the real discussions are happening at the highest levels. According to a report from May by the Corporate Europe Observatory, a list of meetings held by five commissioners with "direct stake in vaccines and medicines," including President von der Leyen, showed a clear pattern of meetings only with pharmaceutical companies and their lobby groups, or with pharma-friendly organizations such as the Bill and Melinda Gates Foundation.

It was thus a disappointment but not a surprise to Botenga and others when the Geneva Health Files recently revealed a confidential communication from the commission showing a bad-faith approach to waiver negotiations that misrepresented the parliament's strong support. The European Union also introduced its own proposal at the WTO in June, which, according to activists, simply reiterates existing flexibilities; many therefore view it as a diversionary tactic to delay talks on the waiver.

Meanwhile, while the chancellor was in Washington, German Health Minister Jens Spahn was reiterating Germany's strong anti-waiver position in Geneva. "I am sure that next year, we will have a surplus of production," Spahn told members of the World Health Organization. To global health activists, this laissez-faire attitude in the midst of a global health crisis of this magnitude is untenable. Spahn, however, like many opponents of the waiver, claims that it is technological know-how, not freeing up patents, that will increase production and availability of vaccines.

The Push for Manufacturing

Yet, as Doctors Without Borders' Dimitri Eynikel explained, this is a false choice. Activists are well aware that the waiver alone will not deliver the necessary vaccine doses. But pressure on the waiver can be maintained while activists also push for the necessary tech transfer. In the United States, a group of American health and humanitarian organizations have called on President Biden to implement a global manufacturing program as part of his 2022 budget. Biden could use the Defense Production Act, Bayh-Dole Act or other legislation, as Public Citizen has argued, to "scale up manufacturing, license patents and know-how to the World Health Organization's Technology Access Pool."

Biden has already employed the Defense Production Act to allow Merck to produce Johnson & Johnson's vaccine. Globally, the World Health Organization plans to set up production hubs around the world, and, on June 21, announced the first hub in South Africa. On July 21, Pfizer announced an agreement with South African company Biovac for production of its vaccine. Yet activists emphasize that, despite the company touting this move, this is a type of license that does not actually provide the South African manufacturer with independent ability to produce the vaccine.

Brook Baker has suggested that the Biden administration could use the threat of the waiver, in the meantime, to bring pharmaceuticals to the table. According to intellectual property law and medicines policy expert Ellen 't Hoen, countries that have financed the development of vaccines should be the ones truly pushing companies to transfer their technology. This means the United States, which contributed almost a billion dollars in public funding to Moderna, Germany, which contributed to the Pfizer/BioNTech vaccine, and the U.K., with its support for the Oxford/AstraZeneca vaccine.

Meanwhile, activists are hoping that pharmaceuticals could still be compelled to transfer know-how and technology to the WHO's COVID-19 Technology Access Pool. During the AIDS pandemic, government pressure became intense enough, according to Baker, that pharma came to the table and began providing voluntary licenses under threat of further government action.

A Reason for Optimism

Despite the obstacles facing the movement, Eynikel said that he feels some optimism, in part because of strong levels of awareness and engagement in the United States. But it's not just there. "My impression for lower and middle-income countries is that they are in it for the long haul," he explained. "They want structural change now. This debate won't go away anymore. I think that's something that high-income countries, including European Union member states, still haven't realized yet."

This was echoed by Baone Twala, a legal researcher at Section 27 in South Africa. "This is extremely reminiscent of the AIDS pandemic when it first began," she explained via e-mail. "However, the difference here is that the South African government has adopted a more proactive approach which is commendable."

Activists in the Global South have been heavily involved since before the waiver was introduced. They've written letters of appeal to the European Commission, to missions, embassies and world leaders; they've also organized protests in front of embassies of countries opposing the waiver.

It is unconscionable that—with only about 1 percent of Africans fully vaccinated and death rates soaring on the continent—pharmaceutical executives have been caught discussing how they can, instead, boost profits in the Global North by raising prices from approximately $19.50 per person for the current round of doses to $150-175 per person for booster shots.

As Eynikel points out, we have, over the course of the pandemic, asked many companies to make important sacrifices to protect our health, including shutting down completely for periods of time. Why, then, "can't we ask the same of the pharmaceutical industry, the companies who have the tools to end the pandemic for everybody, everywhere?"

With the WTO TRIPS Council in recess for summer, activists in Europe expect activities to quiet down until September, when the council reconvenes. These meetings, as well the World Health Assembly at the end of November, will present renewed opportunity for activism around the issue. Meanwhile, in the United States, where activists are reviving pressure on their own government, President Biden's top vaccine diplomat, Gayle Smith, told the Financial Times on Wednesday that she was urging U.S. vaccine makers "to support the development of low-cost manufacturing hubs overseas."

Activists in the United States welcomed the move. In a statement from Public Citizen, Peter Maybarduk, director of the organization's Access to Medicines Program, stated: "We are heartened by Coordinator Smith's support for regional production hubs." But some warn that, despite this positive step, there is still much work to do. "I'm afraid the administration will need to intervene much more forcefully to achieve the knowledge sharing that's needed to end the pandemic," Arthur Stamoulis said.

The question, when it comes down to it, therefore remains, as Eynikel put it: "Can the government go against private interests to protect the public interest?" Activists are holding out hope that, with the Delta variant wreaking havoc and the broken promise of global vaccine equity becoming ever more glaring, the answer to that question might, against all odds, still be a "yes."

Periodical and Internet Sources Bibliography

The following articles have been selected to supplement the diverse views presented in this chapter.

Seth Berkley and Michael Anderson, "How Innovative Financing Will Help Prepare for Future Pandemics," World Economic Forum, April 7, 2022. https://www.weforum.org/agenda/2022/04/pandemic-preparedness-innovative-finance/.

Daniel C. DeSimone, M.D., "Covid-19 Variants: What's the Concern?" Mayo Clinic, March 31, 2022. https://www.mayoclinic.org/diseases-conditions/coronavirus/expert-answers/covid-variant/faq-20505779.

Emma Farge, "Explainer: How the World Health Organization Might Face Future Pandemics," Reuters, February 24, 2022. https://www.reuters.com/business/healthcare-pharmaceuticals/how-world-health-organization-might-face-future-pandemics-2022-02-24/.

Karen Feldscher, "A Prescription for Future Pandemics," Harvard T.H. Chan School of Public Health, March 2, 2022. https://www.hsph.harvard.edu/news/features/a-prescription-for-future-pandemics/.

Taylor McNeil, "How Viruses Mutate and Create New Variants," TuftsNow, June 9, 2021. https://now.tufts.edu/2021/06/09/how-viruses-mutate-and-create-new-variants.

Carrie MacMillan, "Virus Variants: What Do You Need to Know Now," Yale Medicine, February 18, 2021. https://www.yalemedicine.org/news/coronavirus-variants.

Chris Meserole, "How Misinformation Spreads on Social Media—and What to Do About It," Brookings, May 9, 2018. https://www.brookings.edu/blog/order-from-chaos/2018/05/09/how-misinformation-spreads-on-social-media-and-what-to-do-about-it/.

Martin Van Nieuwkoop and Monique Eloit, "We Must Invest in Pandemic Prevention to Build An Effective Global Health Architecture," World Bank Blogs, May 12, 2021. https://blogs.worldbank.org/voices/we-must-invest-pandemic-prevention-build-effective-global-health-architecture.

Kari Paul, "A Systemic Failure: Vaccine Misinformation Remains Rampant on Facebook, Experts Say," *Guardian*, July 21, 2021. https://www.theguardian.com/technology/2021/jul/21/facebook-misinformation-vaccines.

Peter Ramjug, "Vaccine Misinformation on Social Media Can Be a Life-Or-Death Problem," News@Northeastern, January 20, 2022. https://news.northeastern.edu/2022/01/20/vaccine-misinformation-social-media/.

Saswato Ray, "What Vaccine Misinformation Really Tells Us," Harvard Political Review, August 28, 2021. https://harvardpolitics.com/vaccines-social-media/.

Divyah Shah, "What is a Variant? An Expert Explains," Wellcome, November 29, 2021. https://wellcome.org/news/what-variant-expert-explains.

Peter Suciu, "Spotting Misinformation on Social Media Is Increasingly Challenging," *Forbes*, August 2, 2021. https://www.forbes.com/sites/petersuciu/2021/08/02/spotting-misinformation-on-social-media-is-increasingly-challenging/?sh=593922912771.

For Further Discussion

Chapter 1

1. What might be the motivation for some experts to downplay the idea of natural immunity and continue pushing for vaccination for most people? Explain.
2. At the height of polio, 3,000 children died compared to almost 1 million from COVID-19 (as of April 10, 2022, according to the CDC). And yet people flocked to get vaccinated from polio as opposed to the COVID-19 vaccination. What might account for the disparity?
3. How does risk come into play when addressing vaccine safety? Why should it matter?

Chapter 2

1. One viewpoint author writes that most people in the U.S. comply with vaccination protocols but don't speak up about it on social media. How could this affect the rhetoric surrounding vaccines on social media platforms?
2. Many parents interpret information on social media as being equivalent to medical information coming from the CDC. Is this misguided thinking? How might this affect public health?
3. Immunization opponents have used a variety of techniques to convince media users of false information. Have you encountered such tactics on social media? What have you done?

Chapter 3

1. According to some, people have been confused by a barrage of information about the COVID vaccine, and this has led to vaccine mistrust. What should people do about this situation?
2. Some major religions are on record saying that they support vaccination. Should religion play a role in deciding health matters for people other than individuals?
3. Some political leaders have been outspoken about getting the COVID-19 vaccine. Should more well known people such as celebrities and sports figures support vaccination in a public health crisis? Why or why not?

Chapter 4

1. Should vaccines be mandatory? Use facts from the viewpoint articles to back up your argument.
2. Have you heard of the natural immunity theory posed by anti-vaccine believers? How could this anti-scientific view pose a threat to public health?
3. Does social media have a stake in vaccine related issues? What can or should social media do in this area?

Organizations to Contact

The editors have compiled the following list of organizations concerned with the issues debated in this book. The descriptions are derived from materials provided by the organizations. All have publications or information available for interested readers. The list was compiled on the date of publication of the present volume; the information provided here may change. Be aware that many organizations take several weeks or longer to respond to inquiries, so allow as much time as possible.

Bill & Melinda Gates Foundation

500 Fifth Avenue North, Seattle, WA 98109
(206) 709-3100
email: https://www.gatesfoundation.org/about/contact/write-to-us
website: https://www.gatesfoundation.org/

The Bill & Melinda Gates Foundation has a huge presence around the world. Witness work being done globally and read all about vaccine work.

Centers for Disease Control and Prevention (CDC)

1800 Clifton Road NE, Mail Stop D-72, Atlanta, GA 30333
(800) 232-4636
email: https://wwwn.cdc.gov/dcs/contactus/form
website: https://www.cdc.gov/

The CDC is the leading scientifically based organization in the United States and sees as its mission one to protect the health of U.S. citizens. Besides having a robust site containing reliable information, they have online publications including one on emerging infectious diseases.

Eco Health Alliance

520 Eighth Avenue, Suite 1200, New York, NY 10018
(212) 380-4460
email: https://www.ecohealthalliance.org/contact-form
website: https://www.ecohealthalliance.org/

Eco Health Alliance is a global nonprofit agency that works to protect wildlife and public health from the emergence of disease. Read about efforts to promote conservation and by this prevent pandemics and disease.

Immunization Action Coalition

2550 University Avenue West, Suite 415 North, St. Paul, MN 55114
(651) 647-9009
email: admin@immunize.org
website: https://www.immunize.org/

The Immunization Action Coalition's online site contains a vast amount of information about the safety of vaccines. Access a large amount of trustworthy information about vaccines, both in article form and different publications available to print.

Save The Children

501 Kings Highway East, Suite 400, Fairfield, CT 06825
(800) 728-3843
email: supportercare@savechildren.org
website: https://www.savethechildren.org/

Save the Children is an organization dedicated to giving all children a healthy start in life. Find information about what affects children including health issues.

The Task Force For Global Health

330 W. Ponce de Leon Ave., Decatur, GA, 30030
(404) 371-0466
email: info@taskforce.org
website: https://www.taskforce.org/

The Task Force For Global Health has a mission to eliminate the world's worst diseases. Stay informed about the world's deadly diseases and the efforts to control them. Get reliable information and sign up for their newsletter.

The World Bank

1818 H. Street, NW Washington, DC 20433
(202) 473-1000
email: https://www.worldbank.org/en/about/contacts
website: https://www.worldbank.org/en/home

The World Bank sees its mission as two important goals: to end extreme poverty and to support shared prosperity on a global scale. Pandemics and disease with associated health costs are a global crisis which this organization works to aid.

U.S. Food & Drug Administration (FDA)

10903 New Hampshire Avenue, Silver Spring, MD 20993-0002
(888) 463-6332
email: https://www.fda.gov/about-fda/contact-fda#centers-and-offices
website: https://www.fda.gov/

The FDA is responsible for protecting the health of U.S. citizens by monitoring the safety of human and veterinary drugs, medical devices, biological products and much else. Find an almost endless supply of reliable, scientific information about vaccines here.

World Economic Forum (WEF)

350 Madison Avenue, 11th Floor, New York, NY, 10017
phone
email: https://www.weforum.org/contact-us/home
website: https://www.weforum.org/

The World Economic Forum is an international organization that dedicates itself to a public-private cooperation on a global scale. Watch videos and read articles dedicated to cover globally important issues. Look at information that marks World Immunization Week.

World Health Organization (WHO)

1 Dag Hammarskjold Plaza, 885 Second Avenue, 26th Floor,
New York, NY 10017
(646) 626-6060
email: whonewyork@who.int
website: https://www.who.int/

The WHO is the United Nations agency dedicated to global health and safety, and promotes health for all across the globe. Stay informed through articles and videos about current health topics of concern, including interesting news about current research leading to new vaccines.

Bibliography of Books

John Allen. *Vaccine Wars: When Science and Politics Collide.* San Diego, CA: Reference Point Press, Inc., 2022.

Jonathan M. Berman. *Anti-Vaxxers: How to Challenge a Misinformed Movement.* Cambridge, MS. 2020.

Don Brown. *A Shot in the Arm!* New York, NY: Amulet Books, 2021.

Nina Burleigh. *Virus: Vaccinations, The CDC, and the Hijacking of America's Response to the Pandemic.* New York, NY: Seven Stories Press, 2021.

Kristen A. Feemster. *Vaccines: What Everyone Needs to Know.* New York, NY: Oxford University Press, 2018.

Maya J. Goldenburg. *Vaccine Hesitancy: Public Trust, Expertise, and the War on Science.* Pittsburg, PA: University of Pittsburg Press, 2021.

Tara Haelle. *Vaccination Investgation: The Science and History of Vaccines.* Minneapolis, MN: Twenty-First Century Books, 2018.

Peter J. Hotez. *Preventing the Next Pandemic: Vaccine Diplomacy in a Time of Anti-Science.* Baltimore, MD: Johns Hopkins University Press, 2021.

Jill Keppeler. *Fake News.* New York, NY: Rosen Publishing, 2021.

Heidi Larson. *Stuck: How Vaccine Rumors Start and Why They Don't Go Away.* New York, NY: Oxford University Press, 2020.

Dave Levitan. *Not a Scientist: How Politicians Mistake, Misrepresent, and Utterly Mangle Science.* New York, NY: W. W. Norton & Company, 2017.

Michael Miller. *Fake News: Separating Truth from Fiction.* Minneapolis, MN: Twenty-First Century Books, 2018.

Don Nardo. *How Vaccines Changed the World.* San Diego, CA: Reference Point Press, 2019.

Cindy L. Otis. *True or False: A CIA Analyst's Guide to Spotting Fake News.* New York, NY: Feiwel & Friends, an Imprint of Macmillan Publishing Group, LLC. 2020.

Paige Polinsky. *Vaccines: A Graphic History.* Minneapolis, MN: Lerner Publishing Group, 2022.

Marisa Reichardt. *A Shot at Normal.* New York, NY: Farrar Strauss Giroux Books for Young Readers, 2021.

Rebecca Rissman. *The Vaccination Debate. Minneapolis, MN: Essential Library, 2016.*

Index

G

H

I

J

K

L

M

N

O

P

Q

R

S

T

V

W

Y

Z